SO...THAT'S WHY I'M BONKERS!

SO...THAT'S WHY I'M BONKERS!

A girl's guide to surviving the menopause

One woman's journey through menopause, middle age and madness:
Through anecdotes, research and a recently revived sense of humour.

Sheila Wenborne

ISBN-13: 9781518801464
ISBN-10: 1518801463
Library of Congress Control Number: 2015920386
CreateSpace Independent Publishing Platform
North Charleston, South Carolina

Introduction:

decided to write this book after receiving countless emails and phone calls from fellow menopause sufferers asking for advice. This unusual and quite unexpected interest in me came after I was featured in several national newspapers reporting on how I had turned my life round and started a new business as a direct result of my refusal to accept the "Change" as surrender to "old age."

In the following pages, I have tried to present the facts and suggest ways of coping with the menopause. Whether you decide to go down the HRT route or take a more holistic approach to dealing with this often turbulent time of life, as John Lennon once said, "Whatever gets you through the night," is fine.

I hope you will find this book both informative and entertaining but most of all, I hope you find it Inspiring. "Come on Girl! You ain't finished yet!"

If I can be of any further help just yell and I'll hear you. I've probably got all the windows open. ☺

Love

Sheila

www.sheilawenborne.com

I would like to dedicate this book to my husband Joe who has borne the brunt of my bad temper more than once. Without him I would be lost.

Also to my Mum who has always been a silent rock. She never ever complained about my mood swings, finding things in peculiar places or the freezing temperature of our home.

Table of Contents

My Name is Sheila and I'm Menopausal

Of course it wasn't going to happen to me. I was far too young and vibrant to even entertain the idea of walking through the sands of the menopausal desert – that 'thing' that turns many women of substance into gibbering wrecks, incapable of anything more challenging than eating ham straight from the fridge because they're just too tired to make a sandwich.

OK, I was approaching fifty and just a little bit grumpy. But then you would be, working full out as costume designer for a panto company. The hairs on my chin had been coming through at a more regular pace than I could cope with and were stiffer than they once were. But, hey, that's what tweezers were made for. Having said that, failing sight meant I couldn't always see them close-up and it would be down to my husband to point out the rogue offenders, often not realising the beardy growths were actually attached to me.

'Ooh, look. You've got a hair on your face,' he'd say, giving it a tug which would be closely followed by a loud 'ouch' from me and a look of embarrassment from him. On a good day he would get away with a glare. On a bad day I suspect he genuinely feared for his life, and possibly others. The dogs would slouch off and curl up tightly, with the heads under their paws, for fear of making eye contact.

But I was still hot. Admittedly, not always when I wanted to be and sometimes when it was totally inconvenient. Like in the middle of the night when I'd only just got off to sleep after waking, as usual, at 3am for no particular reason. Running around naked with the window open at this time was initially mistaken for some kind of sexual ritual.

'I might be naked and bending over the bed making loud panting noises, but now is not a good time. I'm just trying to stretch out the cramp in my lower back.'

By about 5am I'd be back asleep; until I needed to pee. So it would be up again, awake, with the added extra of a little bit of anxiety. The type that makes you wonder what you're worried about and you worry because you can't remember. Then you worry that you're losing your memory so you go to get a drink of water only to get into the kitchen to forget why you're there.

Still I wasn't prepared to admit that it was possible, if only slightly, that good old Mrs Oestrogen had left the building – and wasn't coming back. I'd fight to keep every last scrap of the very same hormones I hated as a teenager.

Those which had forced their way in and showed real determination to stay for many decades, had upped and left with no warning.

Actually, that's a lie. There was warning and, looking back, probably plenty of it. Someone once mentioned to me that I might be going through the 'peri-menopause'. When they explained what they meant all I could think of was 'dry run'. And that just about sums it up. Everything in the lady garden area had dried up. The thought of sex was about as exciting as doing a VAT return, only without the laughs. Occasionally when it occurred to me I really ought to allow myself to be 'bothered' by my very patient and far more enthusiastic husband, I needed a good week's notice and a run-up. Then I just hoped it would be over before I either a) fell asleep through exhaustion or b) started to sweat, but not in a good way.

At first I didn't want to tell anyone about these peculiar changes to my body – and mind. Maybe the symptoms would pass and were to do with something else? I was tired, been drinking too much, not had enough zinc in my diet and perhaps needed a holiday? Perhaps it was just a 'mini-pause' rather than the full blown menopause. Something I could get over quickly while continuing life with most of my hormones intact?

It was only when one of my slightly younger friends virtually stripped off in an exercise class – before we'd even started moving – asking 'is it hot in here, or is it me?' that I realised I was not alone. Others were shrined in their hoodies and jogging bottoms, hugging themselves close for fear of shivering to death while Mary, my apparently menopausal friend, was considering whether it would be reasonable to do Zumba barefoot, in just her pants and a sports bra (the latter being essential because the general laxity of her bosoms had increased dramatically in recent months).

I've had similar issues with the heating. Windows thrown open in genuine appreciation of fresh air while simultaneously watching my husband's nose turn very slightly blue, even after the application of his particularly thick and versatile Norwegian knit fleece, suggested that my own personal thermostat wasn't to be relied on.

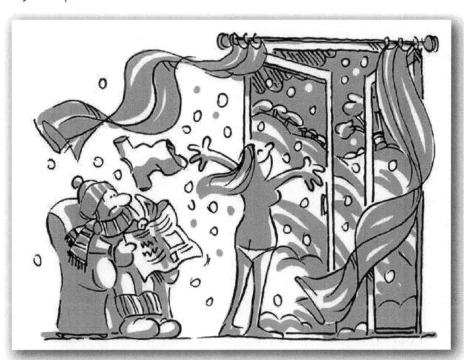

❖ *In ancient times, human beings believed that because a woman did not bleed for nine months before giving birth, infants developed from retained menstrual blood. Menstrual blood, called wise blood, took on powerful meanings. It was used for healing, to fertilise crops and to impart wisdom. It followed that when a woman didn't bleed for a year and had no more children, it was because she retained her wise blood. It was then that she became a respected elder, judge, teacher, healer and leader. Her community respected her power.*

There were other signs that change was upon me. As Deepak Chopra said; 'All great changes are preceded by chaos.' And how absolutely accurate that statement is. Using a mobile phone while simultaneously looking for it in my bag is quite chaotic, just as putting on some rice for lunch only to then go and have a lie down – to wake up to the sound of the smoke alarm as said rice incinerates on the stove.

Life was certainly getting chaotic. I tried to keep busy but failed through a sudden inability to multi-task. It was all I could to do to keep up with the constant sheet changing and application of deodorant to think of anything more challenging.

At that point it was the realisation that whatever was going on was having an impact on my mind as well as my body.

Anatole France is quoted as saying: 'all changes, even the most longed for, have their melancholy; for what we leave behind us is a part of ourselves; we must die to one life before we can enter another.'

That's just about how it felt – like dying, slowly, but not terminally. Just that something was going but I couldn't remember what. My get up and go and had got up and gone.

Thoughts like that would make me cry. Just as the John Lewis advert did at Christmas, and a soppy love song on the radio - and a squashed squirrel in the roadside. Everything was having an impact on me in a very different way.

Nothing else could explain it. There was only one absolute certainty: It was all to do with the M word.

I was going Mad.

ALL CHANGE

I went to the doctor's and asked some questions. I wanted to know why I was getting fat and didn't want sex anymore.

He told me to talk to my husband, then go out and buy a book on the menopause and some bigger knickers.

Well, how Bridget Jones' style underwear was going to resolve the menace of creeping asexuality beat me, so I left with a terrible feeling of having got to the end of the road before I'd finished my journey.

There was nothing else for it. A shopping trip followed by a glass of wine with some girlfriends.

The shopping trip didn't last very long. After an uncomfortable fight with a pair of spanks (how you are supposed to get those things on without pliers and three armies of helpers, I don't know) and a sweaty argument with the non-sweaty, twenty year old sales assistant about the possibility I could be a size 16 rather than a 14, I stormed off to the wine bar and consoled myself with three very swift glasses of Sauvignon Blanc.

By the time my friends had arrived – two of them late because one had forgotten we were meeting and the other one couldn't find her keys (they were in the fridge) – I was asking the bar staff if they could please turn off the heating that was obviously placed behind my back and under my chair.

Very patiently they explained there was no heating and in fact other customers were feeling the cold. (They need one of those Norwegian jumpers).

My friends, experienced in such arguments, suggested that maybe it was the menopause that had brought on my flush.

'Or maybe it's the wine?' said Amelia, in recognition of my denial.

'Don't blame the wine!' I shouted. 'It's the only thing that helps!'

RESOLUTION

After three weeks of solitude, brought on partially by friends being a little bit scared to talk to me, a husband who thought it best not to say anything for fear of reprimand and incredibly painful boobs brought on by the, otherwise seemingly ineffectual HRT, I had a light bulb moment.

It involved trying to turn on a lamp in my office and getting very angry that it wasn't working. I changed the plug, checked the fuse and then finally went to Ikea and bought another one.

My husband was hesitant about querying the new purchase but couldn't contain himself. I explained as carefully as I could that: 'the bloody thing wasn't working. OK?!'

He didn't say anything, just retrieved the old lamp from where I'd rammed it in the kitchen bin, plugged it in and put in a new light bulb.

Then there was light.

I wanted to laugh out loud, but was frightened I might wet myself.

It was far too difficult for me to say sorry because I didn't feel it at all. What I did feel, however, that it was totally wrong for woman – and those around them – to put up with feeling like they've been taken over by aliens.

Something had to be done – and soon.

The Menopause: What is it?

The menopause may not be the best topic of conversation at every dinner party, or supermarket queue, but it's definitely the subject of many a discussion among women who have decided they can no longer remain quiet about something that has come along and hit them like a train in a tunnel.

There are a few who have taken their struggles with navigating the symptoms of menopause to the masses, in the form of blogs and diary pieces on the internet. But it still doesn't form a main item on many media agendas.

So it would seem that anyone who has been taken by surprise by the vagaries of hormonal demise has joined a private club, one that isn't fully documented; a bit like the Freemasons.

Until recently there has been no need within the health service to define what the menopause is. However, The National Institute for Health and Care Excellence (NICE) has now defined a range of guidelines which are available to the medical profession.

The Guideline Development Group comprised experts in menopause and post-reproductive care who were given the brief to respond to the fact that information and support available has been variable and inadequate.

The 'diagnosis and management of the menopause' guidelines will encompass:

- Menopausal women (covering peri-menopause and post-menopause)
- Women with premature ovarian insufficiency (regardless of cause)

Clinical issues to be incorporated:

- Diagnosis and classification of the stages of menopause
- Optimal clinical management of menopause-related symptoms
- Contribution of HRT in preventing long-term potential associated conditions of the menopause (especially osteoporosis and cardiovascular disease)
- Diagnosis and management of premature ovarian insufficiency

Women meet in exclusive places such as changing rooms, usually while wafting themselves following a post-workout flush, or while out walking dogs, and secretly discuss various symptoms they're getting.

Depending on what age it starts, of course, the conversations are fairly humorous.

'Oh, another hot flush, must be my age,' I'd say as I dismissed the feeling I'd been set alight by a stray firework. 'At least it doesn't matter that I've forgotten my coat'

But then it gets more serious. Three months in of no sleep, anxiety attacks and palpitations and people stop thinking they're going through the menopause. They actually think they're dying.

Terrified of the doctor, in case they find something that confirms that suspicion, they start looking on the internet. They're too young for the actual menopause – after all we were all just having a joke about flushes but it was probably the wine, or the double espresso, or stress. Never our age…

It was in 1812 (also famous for that Overture), that the term 'menopause' was first used by the French physician, C P L de Gardanne. Mon dieu!

It's then that the horror begins. The tales of woe, the end of our reproductive life and some pretty fine physical and emotional issues to deal with.

According to the great oracle that is Google, our genetic make-up can influence what happens to us in menopause.

For example, for many people their health and lifestyle when our mothers were pregnant with us (when our eggs were being made) can have an impact as can the nutrition and environment we had growing up.

Seeing as many mothers I've heard about from previous generations enjoyed her gin-filled, smoky weekends and a variety of saturated fats in the guise of fish and chips or roast dinners, it's amazing anyone's eggs appeared at all.

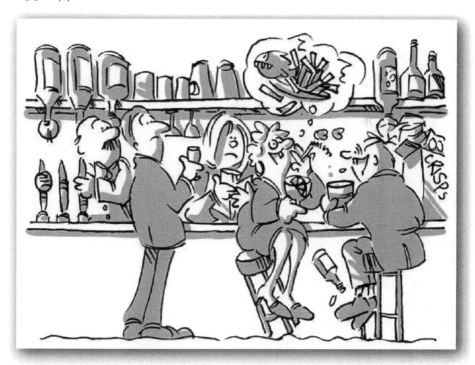

In terms of my own mother, she was always very happy, healthy and active. Whatever happened with her menopause she breezed through it – making it even more of a shock when my symptoms appeared from nowhere.

Add to that the age of first pregnancies, how many there have been and the gaps between them as well as our own health and lifestyles and there's a series of ingredients that can produce a different recipe for all of us.

Research has shown that there are also other influences on peri-menopause symptoms such as level of education, our job, financial and social status and levels of stress.

Education for many was a combination of stress, confusion and soaring sexual interest which lasted from Reception to Graduation. Jobs for most people are a requirement and it is interesting to wonder how they affect one's mid-life responses. Do midwives have a better time of it, being so 'up close and personal' to fertility on a daily basis? If so, how do funeral directors fare?

I spent much of my life running pantomimes. So you'd think I'd have this menopause lark sorted...

'It's behind you!'...

'Oh no it isn't - I'm smack in the middle of it!'

Snow White's dwarves could be Grumpy, Sweaty, Itchy, Ratty, Sleepy, Forgetful and Scary?

So what actually is the menopause? That period, or lack of it, sometimes referred to as the "change of life"?

Put bluntly, as most medical explanations are, it is the end of fertility. It's when our ovaries stop producing an egg every four weeks. According to the NHS it is a time when a woman no longer has monthly periods. They very kindly point out that it is also a time when a woman is unlikely to get pregnant. For anyone who'd stopped reading at that point, they might just wonder whether those odds were based on our bodily functions or the fact that most pregnancies require some kind of physical contact with a member of the opposite sex (unlikely, in the circumstances, really).

In the UK, the average age for a woman to reach the menopause is 51. Some women, however, experience the menopause in their 30s or 40s. Should that be the case then doctors will very kindly refer to you as 'premature' when it comes to the change. As if they hadn't already worked that out.

The hot flush, usually accompanied by sweating, is said to be the most common symptom encountered. It is experienced by over 80% of women and the problem arises as changes in hormone levels upset the temperature regulating part of the brain.

Of course we are likely to blame sudden changes in room temperature, eating spicy foods and stress – although all of these can exacerbate the issue.

❖ *The menopause is probably the least glamorous topic imaginable; and this is interesting, because it is one of the very few topics to which cling some shreds and remnants of taboo. A serious mention of menopause is usually met with uneasy silence; a sneering reference to it is usually met with relieved sniggers. Both the silence and the sniggering are pretty sure indications of taboo. Ursula K. Le Guin*

The other more common symptoms include weight gain and mood swings although it would be understandable that the mood swings come from the weight gain. Standing on the scales and registering another two kilos for no apparent reason is enough to make me feel as low as a snake's belly.

Some self-help sites on the internet say low mood during the menopause is not helped by the fact that this phase of life can be associated with children leaving home, creating 'empty nests' – although personally I feel many women welcome the freedom to flop down at the end of the day without worrying about who has clean clothes, or done their homework.

'I didn't mind the empty nest so much,' said my former colleague, Anna. 'It meant I had more time to myself and didn't have to try and put on a happy face when I was feeling particularly irritated. Although on a deeper level I did feel a bit useless, particularly if I thought of what was happening physically to my body. I can see how some people put the empty nest in the same category as losing fertility and then feeling a loss in terms of femininity.'

Thankfully the inability to hold a thought for no longer than a goldfish can remember its name means that women will forget what is troubling them. It is a known fact that there is a tendency to memory lapses during the menopause. It was explained to me why this happens, but I forget now…

Oh yes, it can happen because of disturbed sleep although it isn't permanent. I managed to get round it by ditching my pride and giving in to post-it notes and lists. My friends who have still failed to buy a diary and rely on their oestrogen-deficient brain receptors often fail to attend meetings and parties – however much they originally thought they would remember both the date and time.

Menstruation can sometimes stop suddenly at this point of life which, at first, might seem like a blessing. However, it's more likely that your periods will become less frequent, with longer intervals between each one, before they stop altogether. So they will catch you out when you least expect it and probably when there's no access to any kind of sanitary product anywhere. It was during some of these situations that the 'Company of Ladies who Use Loo-Roll' first started up and became an accepted tribe among the constantly-taken-by-surprise.

One of my friends has been known to steal the hand towel from a ladies' golf club changing room to deal with her unexpected visitor – unfortunately to the point of regular discussion at committee meetings under the agenda item 'theft'.

Even though it seems like there is no warning to the menopause, all caused by a change in the balance of the body's sex hormones, there is an official term for the months or years prior to the final reality of a barren body.

This lead up is known as the peri-menopause, when oestrogen levels start to decrease, with resulting symptoms that can be shocking to anyone who thought they might have a chance of 'breezing through' their middle years.

At last count there were at least thirty five different symptoms that have been, or can be, attributed to the menopause. Apart from the hot flushes, mood swings, vaginal dryness and murderous personalities, one of my friends – who I will call Melissa – spent three years investigating what she thought was a serious heart complaint (to the point she'd made a new Last Will and Testament and bought as much life insurance as she could without raising suspicion) until a specialist told her that all her palpitations and 'missed beats' were undoubtedly down to a lack of oestrogen.

'He told her it was like driving a car without oil. No wonder I felt so bloody awful,' she said as she tripped down the path of the doctor's surgery, clutching a prescription for HRT.

Of course not everyone needs or suits HRT and the general recommendation is you should only see your GP about menopausal symptoms that are troubling you.

Seeing as there are so many to choose from, I would guess that most would be troublesome. So that's fine advice, as long as you know what symptoms can be related to the change of life, and when they are likely to come along. Few women I know could identify their problems as hormonal immediately. Instead they would complain of digestive disorders, itchy skin, restless legs and a general feeling of malaise. Most would blame their own lifestyles or lack of enough vegetables. It rarely occurred to them to state menopausal changes as a reason.

In women under 50 years of age, the menopause is diagnosed after 24 months without a period. In women aged 50 or over, it's diagnosed after 12 months without a period. In women with a sense of humour it's diagnosed over a few bottles of wine and the general consensus that getting older sucks.

Once of a certain age, we can all join in the discussions. There's no definitive test to diagnose the menopause – apart from a blood test that can sometimes be carried out to measure the level of the follicle-stimulating hormone (FSH). However, no-one really knows what to do with the information once it's received, so is quite often ruled out.

❖ *Women over fifty already form one of the largest groups in the population structure of the western world. As long as they like themselves, they will not be an oppressed minority. In order to like themselves they must reject trivialisation by others of who and what they are. A grown woman should not have to masquerade as a girl in order to remain in the land of the living. Germaine Greer*

And because the list of possible side-effects seems to be endless, everyone can throw something into the general pot of discontent. Whether it is a sudden allergy to hair dye or a persistent wind problem, there's no saying it isn't a shared and uniquely female issue that we all suffer from in varying degrees.

So medical intervention should only be sought if living with the symptoms become unbearable….

Strangely there are relatively few women who seek that help – only about half of the qualifying population - although anyone who is living within shouting distance of any of them might feel they qualify.

The History of the Menopause

Although it has been called many things, there are references to what we now call the menopause spattered through history.

Sigmund Freud, not as revered now as he might once have been, called menopausal women 'quarrelsome' which doesn't seem like a particularly solid scientific appraisal of the mid-life condition.

Fair enough in some ways, as that is probably a true statement - but not helped by the fact he put it in writing and probably said it out loud – and in the hearing of those most affected.

Freud was known to be a great fan of cocaine and suggested the liberal use of drugs, including sedatives, to deal with the effects of hormonal imbalance.

Recent research shows Mrs Martha Freud to be a woman of strong personality who, no doubt taking in her husband's diagnosis, stopped all sexual relationships with her husband after the birth of her sixth child.

Whether or not that was the motivation behind Sigmund's view of women of a certain age is unclear but I know I wouldn't be too happy with any such judgement – particularly when I was ready to pick a fight in an empty room.

At least Mr Freud didn't classify his wife as diseased, as many doctors did in the early eighteenth century.

It was an unwise woman who went to their GP with symptoms of joint pain, deafness, dizziness hot flushes and vomiting. They'd be written off as pretty much on their way out and certainly beyond their usefulness, although slightly nearer to the perfection of a male as no longer being likely to get pregnant.

That all goes back to the classical medicinal definition of women: deformed males; taking away the ability to give birth, by all historic accounts, would make a female closer to 'perfection' by being more like a man.

Well, anyone who has seen the naked male form may have a different view of deformity. (Who else is reminded of the last chicken at the supermarket when their naked partner bends over in front of them?) It's no wonder our predecessors were 'quarrelsome'. I'd be ready to cut off their playthings and stuff them where the sun doesn't shine…

We can be thankful that we have moved a little forward, even if it has taken about three hundred years to get to the point where the NHS is prepared to define the menopause beyond just madness, disease and a pointer to death.

Strangely enough so many women have survived the menopause it has now been proven that is neither a) terminal nor b) catching.

In fact quite a few members of the 'fairer sex' have become experts in the subject – a vast array of older women are listed on The Menopause Exchange as specialists in the field, many of whom have no doubt experienced the effects of hormonal change to varying degrees - and literally are living to tell the tale.

Because of their interest in the subject, and the support of a variety of health professionals, there is now far more information available and considerably more debate – leading to more choice – in how any symptoms are dealt with.

I tried the GP route with varying degrees of success. Although, as you already know I was told by one doctor to buy bigger pants and get on with it, another did provide the opportunity to try HRT. It didn't work for me but I know for many people it does – women who swear they will have to be physically forced to give up those extra hormones they feel so good on them.

Different things work for different people there is no doubt about that – and we are lucky to be in a position to make choices about how to deal with any changes if we have them. There seem to be varying levels of response. Some women sail through the menopause, barely noticing its existence, while others suffer to the point of almost giving up on life – not knowing there is a rational explanation for the fact they basically 'feel crap'.

The Greeks called it 'an imbalance of humours' - which is probably as good an explanation as any, without the knowledge of endocrinology we now have.

I'm sure they were doing their best to help, but this description placed a certain taboo on women worldwide, who then sought to restore their imbalance with means such as leeches, - in the belief the blood-suckers would get rid of the excess blood and recreate balance.

This was because during the Greek times, menstruation was seen as a way for the body to get rid of impurities. So when periods came to a stop, what was thought to happen was that the blood remained within the body, clotting and stagnating.

The solution of the day was the application of leeches — to a woman's genitalia, to her back, or to the nape of her neck.

It must have made shopping very uncomfortable and no wonder it is tradition for middle aged women to go off sex.

'Oh excuse me a minute, I just need to pull that leech off me privates,' isn't what most of us would consider the best start to a night, or even a few minutes, of passion.

At least the Ancient Egyptians went down the route of concocting elixirs to overcome their symptoms.

We call them cocktails these days and many an older woman can be seen stocking up on the gin, vodka and Prosecco supplies for the very same purpose.

There were some strange, no doubt male-dominated, thoughts in earlier years which thought the menopause to be a disorder of the reproductive system, which was then blamed on devoting too much energy to non-reproductive pursuits.

So watch out ladies if you've been watching too much telly, going to Zumba or have a keen interest in Sudoku… your menopause could be blamed on not concentrating on your sexual activity!

The uterus was blamed for a lot of things and often the cure for all ills was a hysterectomy. The word 'hysterical' comes from this, in the belief that all kinds of madness originate from the womb.

For those bringing up teenagers, this may well be seen as the case – on both sides – but pity the poor patient of Isaac Baker Brown who, in 1861, performed a clitoridectomy on her at the age of 57.

The reasons being that: 'for the last year has never slept for more than an hour; always waking with a start; feeling frantic, and very hot and flushed'.

A bit rude, you might think. I don't know about you, but I'm quite fond of my clitoris. It isn't something I think about all the time but I might miss it if it were whipped out during some menopausal high points.

I suppose at the time people didn't realise that this 'change' is only temporary. Yes, menopausal women may fit these old descriptions of: 'sour, egotistical, ugly half-forms with coarse features, moustaches, rough voices and flat chests'; but surely we all feel like that sometimes?

My husband could easily answer to that description after a night out with the lads. What if I decided his 'lack of humour' was offensive enough to cut off his penis? I'm not sure he, or any others from the male race with similar 'symptoms' would be quite so happy to accept this procedure into traditional medicinal cures for a bad attitude.

Not all of the suggestions were quite so drastic. Most of us would probably be OK with the mustard hip-baths, foot baths and 'frictions with stimulating embrocation's' (isn't that a massage?), although perhaps not so with the electric therapy, the filtered juice of guinea-pigs' ovaries, a vaginal plug and iced injections on its removal - or arsenic.

Having said that, a few of my single friends – enjoying the freedom of being in their 50s and knowing exactly what they want – might give a few of those options a go. Internet dating has a lot to answer for...

What does seem to be less radical ideas for dealing with the vagaries of ageing include a good diet, more sleep and possibly golf, although I think that might just be a euphemism for the one rarely mentioned remedy but one that seemed fairly popular: a good orgasm.

I can just imagine popping down to the GP's surgery now to be treated with 'testicular juice' (don't ask) or 'the crushed ovaries of animals'– both popular in the 1930s.

One remedy from the 1700s that stands the test of time, however, is the suggestion of black cohosh – now known as a natural precursor to oestrogen.

Dr Robert Wilson published a book called Feminine Forever in 1966 where he called menopausal women 'castrates' and 'galloping catastrophes'. He said a prescription of oestrogen would make women 'much more pleasant to live with...not dull and unattractive'. He was funded by Wyeth Pharmaceuticals.

Cannabis, opium and belladonna were other favourites, which might explain why so many menopausal women were referred to as 'insane' during their time of change. If they were taking those kinds of remedies it would be more than enough to trigger hysteria.

However, I do have a friend who now has a criminal record for growing her own marijuana. Remembering from her youth how it would make her laugh she thought she would have a go at smoking it – to get her 'humours' back into balance.

Deciding the effect was exactly what she needed she bought some seeds from a reputable website in Amsterdam which made her promise not to cultivate or process the seeds in any way.

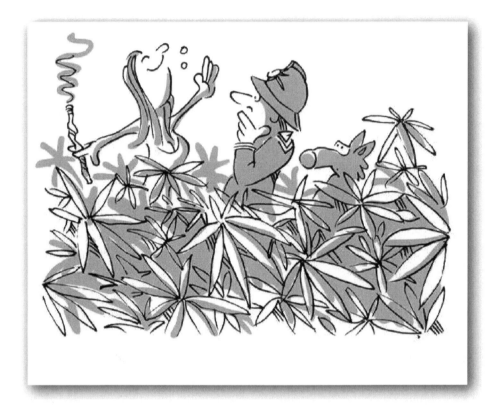

She never reads small print in case it contains something she doesn't agree with, so ticked the box, got the seeds and grew herself 12 plants that did so well the neighbours complained of the smell and reported her to the local CID.

Three police vans, an intensely disinterested German Shepherd and a day in the cells later she was given a caution by a very young CID officer who seemed to accept the mitigation that cannabis was the only solution for her menopausal symptoms.

'He just blushed every time I mentioned it and asked if I was selling it to anyone. I told him, no bloody way. I need every bit of it!'

Amazingly enough it is being considered for a range of other maladies, but not one where a good laugh and the ability to sleep could be all that's needed.

I think she also mentioned that the experience of the police cell – something she welcomed as an opportunity to get away from phones, TV and general life for a few hours – were not unlike the days when women with menopausal symptoms were put away into institutions for the mentally insane on the basis of suffering from 'lunacy'.

The CID officer clearly hadn't studied this part of history and, by her account, looked at her quizzically, no doubt wondering if he could get away with doing the same.

It seems a bit unreasonable to lock your wife up in middle age just because she's not such good company at company at that moment.

If it were a crime to be short-tempered, uncommunicative and not engaged in society then most of the UK's customer service staff would be behind bars.

Tracing the history of more modern day menopausal treatments further back than the early 20th century is difficult since hormones were not officially "discovered" until 1902, by English physiologists Ernest Starling and William Bayliss.

Canadian researcher James Collip made the first breakthroughs in hormone therapy in the 1930s when he extracted an orally active oestrogen from the urine of pregnant women. These were first marketed in the 1940s as a treatment for menopause under the name Premarin.

His discovery led to the development of what is now known as HRT and also bioidentical hormones. HRT treats the menopause with synthetic oestrogens and progesterone while bioidentical hormones are taken from soy or yam plants and engineered in a laboratory.

As the subject started to be taken more seriously, The First International Congress on Menopause was organised in Paris, France in 1976 and from there endocrinology came up with lots more answers.

Apart from offering a chance to control the fluctuation in hormones there were other medical interventions, including aspirin and anti-depressants, that helped relieve symptoms.

Luckily, treatment of menopausal symptoms today is considerably more sophisticated than the remedies of the past. Different forms of HRT and many non-hormonal options are available and huge amounts of anecdotal evidence supports the use of non-medicinal supplements and aids.

As a result we have come a long way from the days of hysteria and since the 1970s the medical acknowledgement of the menopause has been in place – finally liberating middle aged women.

That might explain why a relatively recent survey from the 1980s stated that the vast majority of 8000 women aged between 45 and 55 had no regrets at reaching the menopause. It fact it was younger women who were more concerned about reaching it than those in its midst.

That might have something to do with the more suitable solutions for the symptoms, a greater understanding that the menopause is only a temporary phase of life – and that women are unlikely to be tossed into a cell without their clitoris for the rest of their lives.

Crushed guinea-pig ovaries anyone?

MYTHS OF THE MENOPAUSE

Because the menopause has been shrouded in mystery for so many generations, there are plenty of myths to go around.

The main one is some kind of unwritten rule that you're officially old because it's all started -that you'll be buying a blanket to put over your knees and a Uni Slipper.*

But there are many more which lots of women think are truths, without any real foundation – giving rise to blaming the menopause for everything from a hangover to bunions.

However, as research continues and the 'M' word is allowed more public exposure, the myths are slowly being debunked.

But it is taking time to shake off the stereotypes of the grumpy old woman with no interest in sex and a permanent fixation about the temperature.

A Uni Slipper is designed for both feet to go into one slipper. All fine until you forget you're wearing it and get up to answer the door....

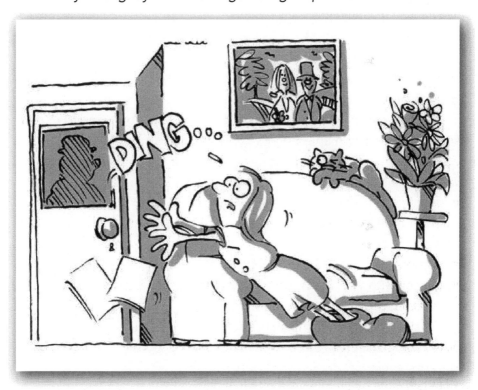

Even men share these false ideas about menopause and may incorrectly assume that a woman is no longer a sexual being after menopause, for instance.

This may well be after a few attempts at physical activity have been thwarted through poor timing – e.g. in the middle of a flush or when extreme fatigue has settled in. But a bit of 'debunking' in terms of what is true, and what isn't, about the menopause should soon overcome those issues.

MENOPAUSE BEGINS AT 50

Well, it could be that your menopause begins at fifty. But your friends' versions might start at 40, 46 or 61. The average is around 52 but it doesn't happen overnight – often it is a gradual onset of symptoms, if you are going to get any at all.

Menopause is technically defined as the absence of a menstruation for a period of one year but with the popularity of the Mirena coil for post-children women, where bleeding stops altogether for the majority, this is difficult to assess.

Also, women sometimes say they didn't know they could start having symptoms many months – or even years - before the onset of menopause. You may even still be having periods when you get the odd hot flush, unusual fatigue, mood swings, irritability, and possible weight gain.

Many of these symptoms could have nothing to do with age and could all be down to a delight in the new flavours of Cadbury's chocolate, various offers on Prosecco at Lidl or Aldi -or just *having* to stay up late to watch episodes of Poldark over and over again (in the interests of historical accuracy, of course).

Yes, the hormones will fluctuate through peri-menopause but poor old oestrogen, progesterone, and testosterone can't be blamed for everything we put our body through.

Stress, as any doctor will tell you, is just as likely to cause these symptoms and for women 'of a certain age' these hormones can be very sensitive to abnormal adrenal function – one of the side-effects of long-term stresses whether they are real or perceived.

So, if you don't like your boss or you're fed up with your next door neighbour's cat puking on your door mat every other day then these factors might be causing some of your symptoms, rather than the menopause itself.

The menopause doesn't mean getting old, either. A woman can expect to live decades past menopause and she will spend a large portion of her life in post menopause – i.e. when it's all over. Despite common opinion (largely from those yet to go through this rite of passage) she can feel healthy, energetic and motivated for many years after the change.

❖ *Women may soon be able to prolong their childbearing years by taking a pill to delay menopause, according to fertility expert, Robert Winston. He recently told the Cheltenham Science Festival that techniques might be developed within a decade to help extend the life of women's eggs. "We think we have identified a protein which might be able to be used to prolong the life of those eggs," he said. "Women are healthier than they were before and the period before menopause could be extended without risk," he said. Lord Winston also said more couples were delaying having babies, leading to problems with fertility. "What we are seeing is increasingly a society where women are ... getting educated and careers in society but their biology is working against them," he said. "In the time you've been listening to me speaking, every woman of child-bearing age in the audience will have lost two eggs," he said, adding: "By contrast, I will have made 150,000 new sperm." Only a man would feel the need to point that out.*

MENOPAUSE IS A DISEASE

One of the biggest misconceptions about menopause is that it is a disease that requires rapid treatment.

For those who have found the symptoms uncomfortable and challenging, they may certainly demand immediate respite – just as anyone might seek help for a backache or skin complaint.

Others may hope that all will pass in good time, but regardless of how each individual approaches this time of their lives; menopause needs to be recognised as normal and natural – and to actively take part in the process. This means accepting the changes, weighing the risks and using treatments where appropriate.

If that means eating an entire Banoffee Pie to yourself while watching repeats of 'Love Actually' then so be it; whatever the needs for requiring that 'treatment', they are as valid as anyone else's.

YOU CAN'T GET PREGNANT

Pregnancy can occur if you are still experiencing menstrual cycles, however irregular*. Some women mistakenly think it can't happen in the peri-menopause, but then there was a time they thought it couldn't happen if you 'did it' standing up.

However, even the weakest cycle means there could be some fertility. A bit like Sainsbury's at 5pm on Christmas Eve. It might look like everything's gone and the shop's about to shut, but there will always be a few eggs hiding in the corner for emergencies.

So, if the timing is right, then fertilization can occur. Health practitioners recommend that an effective birth control method should be used until it has been at least a year since your last period. Garlic and excessive wind can work, although more traditional methods are generally advised.

This requires sexual activity involving a living male.

THERE'S MORE CHANCE OF CANCER

There seems to be more chance of cancer whatever you do. From sniffing creosote (strangely addictive during some hormonal changes, I've heard) to eating the wrong type of margarine, life carries risks.

It is medically true to say that all changes to anyone's body can be a trigger when it comes to increasing the risk of cancer - and so it figures this is also true with the menopause.

Natural drops in protection occur when some hormones deplete – but all is not lost, as the way to combat the risk is to follow a healthy diet by cutting down on sugars, alcohol (only a bit.. there is plenty of anecdotal evidence to suggest a few glasses of good wine here and there can be highly beneficial), wrong types of fats and taking more exercise. The other major factor could be to reduce stress where possible – which is why the warning about not giving up alcohol completely (if you enjoy it) is put forward.

A SALIVA TEST CAN DIAGNOSE THE MENOPAUSE

If you feel like spitting at nature's vagaries – here's your chance! There are some health practitioners who claim your saliva can tell you whether you're depleted in hormones, or not.

However, accurate tests for the menopause are difficult to subscribe whether they are from saliva or blood. The results can be variable because levels vary throughout the day plus the desired levels haven't been established by the medical profession – not least because one woman's experience could be very different to another's, even with the same readings.

MENOPAUSE CAN MAKE YOU MAD

The jury could be out on this one. There seems to be plenty of evidence that women going through the menopause will experience mood swings, but this does not mean you will necessarily turn into a screaming, irrational person.

Try telling that to the screaming, irrational person, who has decided to drive all the way to a shop five miles down the road for something – only to forget what it is they went for. Or realise they have left their purse in the microwave. It is at this point it would be reasonable to assume that menopausal women are mad, even if temporarily.

The raging, hormonal middle-aged woman seems to be the common image, and the butt of many stand-up jokes, but it is generally a false stereotype.

Some of the changes of menopause come around very shortly after the 50th birthday party which, in itself, can leave a few women feeling sad or nostalgic. Some say they might be mourning the passing of their fertile, child-bearing years. Others are more likely to mourn the days when the idea of a party was an exciting one – not one to fear for a) the inability to stay awake after 10.30pm b) the fact that 'party' clothes now look like fancy dress outfits and c) you actually want to invite your parents.

YOU'LL GET FAT

Is it really the menopause that makes some – but certainly not all – middle aged women fat?

According to various experts on the matter, although weight gain can be an issue in menopause that doesn't mean it can't be controlled.

Well, that's what they think. After a lifetime of restriction maybe it is just the time when women think 'sod it' because life's too short not to have a bacon sandwich; or a pub lunch; or tapas with the girlfriends.

After years of staying in on 'school nights' and restricting calorie intake because that is what all the women's magazines suggest, many might just decide that – in the event of a life threatening situation – they might just regret NOT having that piece of cake.

There is the common thought that the cause of any increase in body fat is hormonal fluctuations telling your body to hang on to what it's got, to protect itself. This is something that the older woman can relate to.

'It took me a long time to make this body. It's vintage and valuable. I need to keep it, even if that does mean some form of fat storage around the waist and hips.'

Some may feel the need to restrict calories, take up exercise and generally feel miserable with some vigorous regime to attack the fat.

This isn't necessary and any slimming magazine will show pictures of women in, or past, their menopause and they lose their weight the same way anyone else does - by following a diet based on good nutrition and lower carbohydrates. The science is the same, hormones or not.

There may be a few pounds keener to stay around than they were before, but who can blame them?

YOU'LL GO OFF SEX

You only have to look at older women in the public eye to know that you don't go off sex just because you're a certain age. You might go off it for other reasons of course. Lack of imagination, boredom and something good on the television might be enough to keep you off the boil – just as a bit of imagination and courtship can bring you straight back again!

Although there are some issues in menopause such as vaginal dryness and discomfort with sexual intercourse, a woman's intimacy, bonding and sexual experiences can become more meaningful. A woman can feel, look and act sexy after menopause. In fact some women find that they feel sexier when they don't have to worry about birth control or periods each month.

Although sex can be enjoyable at any age, the general message is that it is normal to experience a decrease in libido. But the fact is that sex is an important part of a relationship and without it, intimacy can be compromised.

So while you might go off the idea of sex because of some symptoms, these can be managed and 'normal service resumed' with a bit of thought and planning. If it continues then discuss the matter with a doctor or health practitioner who might be able to recommend something to help.

❖ *In 1966 the author of "Feminine Forever", Robert A. Wilson, MD, declared the menopause "a natural plague" and menopausal women "crippled castrates." A little harsh by anyone's standards and it's a wonder he didn't end up a crippled castrate himself.*

YOU'LL GET HOT FLUSHES

The caricature of the menopausal woman is one suffering from a massive breakdown in her personal thermometer. It is seen as the first sign that 'the change' is on its way and Mrs Oestrogen is going to be going part-time – with a possible view to retirement.

However, many women don't get them – and if they do will put it down to something else. Like the fact the heating's on too high, something which is easily remedied by turning it down until someone else in the house goes blue.

There is a theory that 'Man in Norwegian Jumper' – a common sight in pubs around the UK during autumn months – has developed because of menopausal women refusing to allow any form of heat in the home. Driven to despair, they have no choice but to dress in the thick woollies as part of their constant bid for warmth.

For those who do get hot flushes, it saves a fortune in clothing and can be very useful when shut outside because you've forgotten your keys again.

YOU'LL STOP HAVING HORMONES

Whatever the medics and cynics might think, hormones might hide but they never really go away.

There may be a slight imbalance and/or decline of hormones, but those ever-present adrenal glands still produce up to half of our oestrogen and progesterone. The levels may drop during our older age but they don't go away completely. So yah, sucks, boo to anyone who thinks otherwise…

MENOPAUSE IS PHYSICAL

One of the most reported symptoms of menopause, other than hot flushes and irregular periods, is a sense of feeling down or blue – sometimes followed by feeling almost manic.

My friend Susan was constantly concerned about something but she didn't know what. She'd leave the house wanting to go home, despite being a very sociable person.

'I just didn't feel quite right about something. It was like I'd always forgotten something or had just had some bad news, but never actually had. It was quite unnerving and not like me at all. It was only when someone explained that changes in hormone levels can produce mood swings that I thought it was all down to the menopause.'

It reminded her of being a teenager, when she'd feel great one minute and fed-up the next. In those days most things were cured by playing the same song over and over again – sometimes ringing 'Dial a Disc' where you could hear the latest Number One down the telephone.

Now Susan just downloads a few songs on iTunes and then tries to work out how to play them on her phone without calling everybody in her phone book and deleting all her recent messages by mistake.

It is like hitting puberty from the other direction and we should all learn to be a little more tolerant of ourselves at this turbulent time.

It's bound to get on your nerves!

HRT IS THE ONLY OPTION

While HRT is a solution for many women, many of whom would swear by it, for some there can be potential risks and side effects.

In my own personal journey I found that HRT caused as many problems as it solved. No-one could get anywhere near me, my breasts were so sore, and I didn't feel the benefit of increased hormones elsewhere.

I decided it wasn't for me although I know there are many women who are now in their 70s and refusing to come off their medication because they feel so good on it.

Like everything else it is a matter of sorting out what works for you. HRT wasn't for me but I was lucky enough to find other methods – in my case, magnetic therapy - totally natural - that did seem to help.

Often women start to help their symptoms with the natural approach, using herbs, vitamins, alternative treatments and products to improve their symptoms. Sometimes it is all they need and often only for a short while.

The main thing is to seek advice from those people you trust and listen to what your body wants. If you think HRT will work and you want to give it a try, find out the risks for you – don't listen to anyone who swears by it or hates it – and then make a decision.

There isn't one rule for all – it is important to do what is right for you.

Menopause around the World

Although menopause is a physical occurrence for all women, albeit in varying degrees, it would be easy to think it is treated the same throughout the world.

Some will say that a woman's experience of the menopause is largely down to personal attitudes and emotions as well as wider factors such as the role and status of women in society.

In some cultures menopausal women don't report, for example, hot flushes. This could be due to dietary patterns or lifestyle although other explanations include the older women and their contribution to society received more recognition – and so aging is viewed positively. Alternatively it could be the case that taboos still exist about openly discussing the symptoms of the menopause and maybe the topic isn't brought up as openly as it is in Western countries.

Interestingly, there's no translation for 'menopause' in some languages. In Japanese the closest word is 'konenki', which describes 'a transition in terms of lived experience', rather than focusing on the woman's body coming to a stop in reproduction.

This doesn't necessarily mean that Japanese women don't experience the menopause, because there periods stop like the rest of us, but they put a different emphasis on the experience. Their culture respects old age and maybe the process of change in mid-life is seen differently.

However, whatever the individual's response to the change – from wanting to repeatedly punch a partner for leaving the cap off the toothpaste, to crying at kittens mewling for their mothers – there is no doubt they can either be side-lined, or buoyed, by cultural and societal responses.

Society can often dictate a woman's perception of themselves - and where ageing is considered to be a loss, then the menopause can offer the first marker along this journey. Alternatively, where getting older is seen as normal and natural, and a time of true freedom, it offers a time of positive change.

Research has shown, for example, that women from Western Europe are more likely to worry about their mental health during the menopause while Arab women are concerned that their partners won't love them or find them attractive any more.

Eastern women tend to weather the storm of thunderous hormones a little more lightly while the Jewish matriarch seems to hardly notice it happening.

So how can that happen? Is it just a cultural thing that turns some Western women into demons with multi-personality disorders while their Eastern counterparts look on with confused amusement?

Could the differing responses really be down to culture? The British have lived in a society that tends to be youth orientated, where the menopause is seen as a loss of everything associated with being young, vital and beautiful. By seeing the change as some kind of degenerative disease, to be conquered and cured or overcome, then it is no wonder so many people find it a challenge.

In studies among Australian women, most claimed to suffer with menopause-related ailments while those in non-Western cultures have an easier time.

THE USA MENOPAUSE

In the USA, women commonly associate menopause with symptoms such as hot flushes and night sweats – so maybe not so different from us although no doubt they do it bigger than us.

However, the SWAN study looked at over 3000 women across the country and found big differences in peri-menopause symptoms depending on the ethnic group the respondents belonged to. The differences observed between African Americans, Hispanic and non-Hispanic Whites and Chinese Americans applied to both types of symptoms and the degree of bother that they caused.

A review of how hot flushes vary around the world showed some big differences: In North America they have been reported as affecting between 30% and 75% of women, and in Europe around 20 - 30%, whereas in Asia the range was from 5 – 20%. In some groups in India nobody reported hot flushes and in Mayan women in Mexico, nobody reported any peri-menopause signs at all, other than menstrual changes

EUROPEAN CULTURES

No-one would expect anything else from the Italians than a totally romantic and sexy view of menopause.

There is a natural 'rite of passage' within their culture. It is seen as the natural next stage and is viewed positively and although Italian women report some physical symptoms, they appear to maintain their self-esteem and sexuality.

Brochures on Tuscany have been appearing on Menopausal Mary's coffee table a lot recently, only marred by the fact they have been sent by Saga.

A Norwegian study followed nearly 2300 women from Hordaland County from 1997 to 2009 and reported problematic symptoms from menopause for four years, on average. Only one per cent of the group reported being plagued by symptoms for as long as twelve years, and just 36 per cent reported daily hot flashes.

BjørnGjelsvik at the University of Oslo, who led the Norwegian study, said that the conclusion was that Norwegian women report less problematic symptoms and have shorter periods with daily hot flushes than US women.

Also their men aren't afraid to wear a thick jumper regardless of the external temperatures and so their wives can alter the temperature controls as much as they like.

EASTERN CULTURE

Now, this is more like it.

In the Japanese culture, menopausal women are revered, seeing as having increased worth and having reached a summit of achievement. As a result it is seen positively – almost like an honour.

In research undertaken by Margaret Lock in 1980, she found that the symptom most likely to be reported by Japanese women during menopause was shoulder stiffness, which seems somewhat peculiar. Perhaps from raising their hands in sheer joy at having got to the top of that mountain called youth, and surviving.

Asian women generally seem to have positive experiences of the menopause, probably because they gain equality with men once menstruation and child-rearing is over. They are seen to be moving towards something else rather than moving away from their role as a younger woman. In a study in Hong Kong, researchers found that joint and muscle problems were the most common symptoms. In all of these studies women reported symptoms as mild.

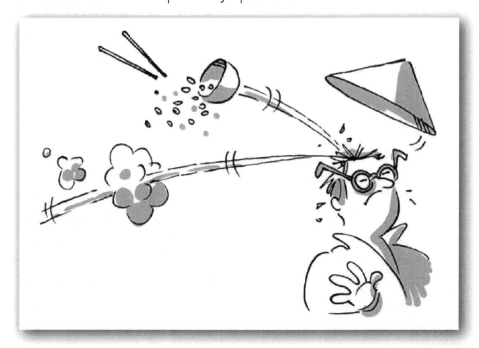

INDIAN MENOPAUSE

Anthropologist, Marcha Flint, first looked at the menopausal experiences of women in non-Western cultures in 1970. She studied 483 women in India and found that most complained of no symptoms during menopause other than changes in their bleeding cycles.

Women, who were veiled and secluded before menopause, could now "come downstairs from their women's quarters to where the men talked and drank home brew" and could publicly visit and joke with men after menopause (Flint 1975).

That would be an interesting concept in modern day Britain. I can't think of many women being particularly keen on the prospect of drinking home brew with male companions. But throw a 'fruit based drink' into the mix and things could become far more fun than solitary confinement.

AFRICAN MENOPAUSE:

We should take note of African women, who view their change as a blessing. Instead of being 'down-graded' by their male counterparts they are seen as equal. Not only are their childbearing responsibilities at an end but they are free for other pursuits. Perhaps their abilities at making home brew are seen to be particularly valuable?

❖ *Spotting or bleeding after Menopause is often viewed as a mark of Witchcraft in Africa*

ANCIENT CULTURES

A comparative study done in the 1980s by Yewoubdar Beyene, looked at Mayan women in a village in the Yucatan, Mexico. She found that no Mayan women reported either hot flushes or cold sweats at menopause.

Whether they did have any symptoms or not might be down to communication. As with the Japanese, Beyene also found that there was no local term for "hot flush or flash" in Mayan culture.

Perhaps they just had to rely on turning the heating down and hoping their husband didn't notice or had the sense to buy a Norwegian jumper.

When Beyene conducted a study of women living in a mountain village on the island of Evia in Greece, she found similar reporting of peri-menopause symptoms as in the rest of Europe and North America.

But is it just culture that shapes our responses to the menopause? Some researchers suggest that lifestyle may play a bigger role than previously thought. We know that hormone levels are largely influenced by how we eat, sleep, and exercise, and many studies have shown a direct relationship between diet and menopause symptoms (for example, Japanese eat a lot of soya yet experience much less, if no, hot flushes).

CULTURE OR SOMETHING ELSE?

So, do British and American women report more symptoms because of stress or the impact of their diet on their hormones, or is it because they live in a culture where the menopause can be treated in the same way as a disease – to be overcome and the symptoms hidden?

What does seem to be clear from all the research is that many women do experience hot flushes at the time of the menopause but whether they are bothered by them will depend on some degree to their culture. Whether they are more bothersome in cultures where women are treated more negatively at this time of life is still a matter of debate.

Dealing with the Symptoms

For some people the first signs of menopause may not be attributed to the change of life.

Indigestion, unusual heart palpitations, general fatigue and insomnia are common complaints among older women.

These can be linked to hormonal changes but may also be a sign of something else – which is why doctors can often by demonised for not recognising the symptoms of the menopause sooner.

Jane is one of my friends who never goes to the doctor yet in a space of three years had presented with signs of IBS, a heart defect, low functioning thyroid, depression, arthritis and general bad mood. It was only after a routine check for something else that someone suggested a hormone check that all the symptoms were linked.

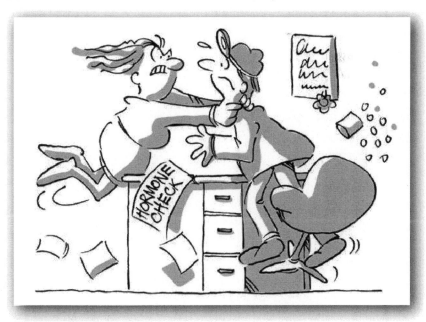

A few weeks later, with the help of some self-help remedies and a low dose of HRT, all the symptoms she'd been complaining about just disappeared.

'I couldn't believe they were linked with each other, or with the menopause. I thought my digestion was shot to pieces because of the years of abuse I'd given it with takeaways and booze – and that my heart was finally suffering because I didn't do my three lots of half hour exercise a week. As for the depression and bad mood, that was because I had constant indigestion that kept me awake, so I didn't sleep and that meant everything ached.'

Often when symptoms are diagnosed as being menopausal, there is the chance of being offered hormone replacement therapy – HRT – which creates differing responses.

Some time ago there was some suggestion that it could increase rates of breast cancer – although now the thoughts are it can be a good choice for some women, with its own benefits in terms of protecting the heart and against some kind of other cancers.

Studies continue to be under review, and it would seem that age and the onset of menopause may play a significant role in determining the best course of treatment. Not all women, nor their symptoms, should be treated in the same way.

BIOIDENTICAL HORMONES

For those who are nervous of synthetic substitutes for our hormones, there are bioidentical versions which are similar in structure to the hormones your body would produce naturally. They are still made in a laboratory so aren't as natural as their name might sound and are, effectively, still drugs.

Many people try alternative methods before committing to a prescription and the first port of call is often dietary changes. A well-balanced diet is essential during the menopause as it enables the body to adjust automatically to the hormone changes, naturally maintaining oestrogen from the adrenal glands and fat deposits.

One area of interest and discussion when it comes to the menopause is that of soya. Eaten in large quantities in the Far East these plant oestrogens seem to have a protective effect as well as being able to help balance the hormones responsible for menopausal symptoms such as hot flushes while also helping to reduce cholesterol.

The best way of gaining these through food would be from eating fermented soya, hops, red clover, sage, alfalfa and flaxseeds.

Not always delicious on their own each can be used as an ingredient, or if you want to get everything in one hit there are many women who swear by a Nutribullet.

'This thing blitzes up all the ingredients for an anti-menopause smoothie in about three minutes' said my friend Yvonne.

A true exponent of all things nutritional and natural she blends up alfalfa and flaxseeds with a variety of fruits and vegetables on a daily basis and reckons it keeps her 'one step away from the madness'.

There are many supplements cited as being beneficial during the menopause. The basic foundation and mantra of a good diet and exercise go as 'read' but add that to some of the following and reports would suggest they could help with a range of symptoms.

VITAMIN C

Vitamin C has a number of benefits at all times of life although giving menopausal women vitamin C with bioflavonoids has been shown to help reduce hot flushes.

It also helps the skin's elasticity by building up collagen which can therefore help with vaginal dryness and problems with the bladder, such as urge or stress incontinence which is common during hormonal changes.

VITAMIN E
This is another vitamin good for flushes and vaginal dryness. Studies have shown that a relatively small amount taken on a daily basis can be helpful.

B VITAMINS
The menopausal symptoms of anxiety, tension, irritability and poor concentration can also be attributed to a lack of Vitamin B and stress. A good supplement will help alleviate the pressure on the adrenal glands at this time.

OMEGA 3 FATTY ACIDS
Fats have had a bad press, particularly when it comes to losing weight but without the essential versions, menopausal women can suffer from a host of symptoms from dry skin and hair to depression, tiredness, breast pain and aching joints. Omega 3 fats also have an anti-inflammatory effect of the body.

MAGNESIUM
Magnesium is another supplement good for dealing with the symptoms of stress such as anxiety, irritability and mood swings. It is also important for bone strength – which at the time of the menopause is an issue because of the increased likelihood of osteoporosis.

CALCIUM
Calcium is often undervalued yet it does so many things in terms of ensuring normal blood clotting, good muscle function plus strong, bones, teeth, nails and hair. It has also been shown that good levels of calcium help with weight loss and proper functioning of the nervous system.

VITAMIN D

Vitamin D is required for calcium absorption, preventing cancer – particularly breast cancer – as well as limiting the risk of type 2 diabetes and osteoporosis. Low levels are associated with rheumatoid arthritis, bowel disease and poor immune function, while it is thought that good levels can slow the ageing process.

HERBS

As well as a variety of vitamins and minerals, many herbs are hailed as the answer to difficult issues throughout the menopause. The main ones are referred to as 'adaptogens', because of their balancing effect on the body.

BLACK COHOSH (CIMICIFUGARACEMOSA)

This is the go-to herb for hot flushes, mood swings and night sweats. It doesn't increase oestrogen levels but offers what is known as selective oestrogen receptor modulators which can stimulate oestrogen receptors in some parts of the body such as the bones and the brain, but not in others.

> ❖ *It might feel like the last thing you want to do when you're breaking out in hot sweats but regular exercise has been shown to help ward off the sudden onset of flushes. A study from Penn State University, US, found that exercise helped almost entirely prevent the onset of hot flushes in the 24 hours after physical activity.*

AGNUS CASTUS (VITEXAGNUSCASTUS)

This herb works on the pituitary gland – the one that tells the ovaries to release hormones – by levelling out hormones if they become too high, or too low. This is particularly helpful in the peri-menopause years because hormones can be fluctuating widely and this herb can create stability.

DONG QUAI (ANGELICA SINENSIS)
Dong quai is an herb from Traditional Chinese Medicine helpful for both the hot flushes and night sweats. It is also helpful for fatigue and disturbed sleep.

SAGE (SALVIA OFFICINALIS)
Another herb useful for controlling both hot flushes and night sweats, it is often taken as a tea.

MILK THISTLE (SILYMARINMARIANUM)
Milk thistle improves liver function, while it is busy detoxing your hormones.

GINKGO BILOBA
Memory problems are a known symptom of menopause and this herb is found to be very useful in terms of improving learning ability, memory and concentration.

SLEEPLESS AND UNSETTLED.
There are very practical solutions to some of the more disruptive menopausal solutions.

When it comes to dealing with the insomnia that so often comes with the peri-menopause, one suggestion is sleeping regular hours with no Sunday sleep-ins. This, according to accepted medical advice, ensures good sleep every night.

All fine to say but if you've had six nights on the trot without little more than two or three hours sleep at a time, Sunday morning (and part of the afternoon) might be the only time in the week you get to have any shut-eye at all. Like all advice, try it to see if it works.

If it doesn't, my view is to sleep where you can and when you can. (Although avoid park benches. It can lead to uncomfortable questions from various authorities. Particularly late at night).

Often the problem of sleeplessness accompanies hot flushes and so if you wear clothing in bed; try to make sure it is made from moisture-wicking fabrics.

OK, I can hear what you are thinking. There's me banging on about not getting any sex, or sleep, and I want you to wear an Andy Pandy outfit at night.

Believe it or not there are fabrics that have been tested on athletes – those sweaty people who regularly do more than their three times a week for half an hour – and by all accounts they keep people dry. They won't stop the night sweats but they might help make them feel more manageable.

It might also go without saying that it helps to keep your bedroom cool. Lower temperatures signals to the body it is time to sleep although if you spot your partner eyeing up his Norwegian jumper pre-bedtime then think about what you might mean by 'cool'.

DOWNWARD DOG

Another method of keeping everything under control without taking any drug of supplement could be yoga, according to researchers who have found that regular practice can limit symptoms of the menopause.

Professor Nancy Woods and colleagues at the University of Washington, Seattle, examined a range of non-drug studies, including herbal medicine, Chinese medicine, yoga, exercise and relaxation. The researchers found that relaxation therapies and yoga showed the most promise.

My friend Anna often did her yoga with her dog, Baldrick. They both enjoyed the 'downward dog' and practiced every morning. That was until the attendant where she walked Baldrick (a large park opposite a primary school) suggested she might like to continue any such future activity in private.

❖ *Yoga practice cut hot flushes by 31% in one study, and other research has found that regularly doing yoga improved libido, mood, and craving control.*

LOTS OF LITTLE PRICKS

In a study published in the journal Menopause, researchers wanted to see how the ancient art of acupuncture affected the regularity and severity of hot flashes a woman experienced while going through natural menopause.

Acupuncture stimulates anatomical points on the body as a form of healing, usually involving the use of thin, metallic needles that penetrate the skin.

The research team looked at twelve studies, involving 869 women between the ages of 40-60 who were going through natural menopause and who underwent various forms of acupuncture.

They found that the women had experienced a reduction in the severity and frequency of hot flushes for up to 3 months, possibly by triggering a response in the nervous system which regulates body temperature.

HYPNOSIS

Another therapy that garnered good results in a recent study is hypnosis, which showed to be an effective treatment for hot flushes which, in a study conducted by researchers at Baylor University's Mind-Body Medicine Research Laboratory, reduced them by as much as 74%.

REFLEXOLOGY

Dating back to Ancient Egypt, reflexology is the practice of treating reflex points and areas in the feet and hands that relate to corresponding parts of the body. Each organ and structure within the body is linked to the feet by energy channels or meridians.

Research carried out at the UK School of Complementary Health in Exeter indicated a marked decrease in anxiety, depression, insomnia, hot flushes and night sweats among menopausal women who received regular reflexology over a 4 month period

It works by helping to restore balance to the endocrine system and calming the central nervous system, which can help with sleep disturbances and anxiety.

If yoga, acupuncture and reflexology seem like a step too far, then another opportunity to test out a natural solution to symptoms is something called 'Mindful Deep Breathing'. This is practiced during yoga and meditation has a proven calming effect on the mind and can ease menopausal anxiety and hot flashes – without having to get down with a dog or salute to the moon.

The suggested method is that as soon as you feel a hot flash coming on; begin by inhaling through your nose to the count of four. Hold your breath for seven counts. Then, exhale completely through your mouth to a count of eight. This is one breath. Try to complete this cycle two more times, but preferably not in the queue for the bank – unless you've learned how to do it quietly.

GADGETS

If you don't want to do anything at all, there are also many gadgets that can help out – handheld fans, cook packs and spray products are on the market to help many a hapless woman suffering with a sudden burst of heat. There are also small devices that can cool skin – or just place a bag of frozen peas against your neck (assuming you are at home and not in the supermarket) can have the same effect.

Again, I can't help but repeat the efficacy of magnets. These days, magnetic therapy is used in one way or another in many areas of conventional medicine – certainly when it comes to hi tech imaging instruments and for promoting the healing of fractures.

If they have this effect on these areas there is every reason to believe that static magnets can have powerful properties in dealing with a range of symptoms associated with menopause.

Whether worn as jewellery or worn in straps or within clothing, static magnets are increasing in popularity and are widely believed to offer therapeutic benefits.

Whatever action you decide to take to deal with the symptoms, there is no doubt that diet and exercise – as ever – will have an impact.

Out of the Ordinary

For some people the change is relatively straightforward. A few hot flushes and irregular periods and then it's all over. Those we call the 'deeply blessed'.

But for some, the symptoms can be both extreme and unusual.

For example, medical studies show that around one per cent of women will suffer from unexplained premature ovarian failure (POF), where the menopause starts before the age of 40 – and up to six per cent will experience premature menopause.

There was a time (pre symptoms) that I would have thought this could be a blessing. With all the trouble I had with periods from my teens until my middle age, the thought of losing any hormones to do with menstrual cycles filled me with glee.

The old adage 'Be Careful What You Wish For' came back to haunt me. As much as I wanted everything to do with my menstruation to be over, I didn't ever anticipate what a trauma losing those damn hormones could be.

EARLY MENOPAUSE

One of the more devastating side effects of premature menopause is infertility, because then the woman can't ovulate to produce her own eggs. The only chance of having a baby is from a donor egg.

There are many possible causes for its development, including autoimmune diseases, cancer treatment and family history, but for some women the causes can remain a mystery.

As unlikely as it might sound when thirteen year old, Amanda, felt bad-tempered and emotional, her family and friends put it down to being a teenager.

Her weight had almost doubled in the space of a few months and no-one had any idea what was going on until she went to the doctor to discover she was going through the menopause – and probably had been since she was just eleven, and a time when all she should have been worrying about is periods and the onset of spots.

However spots are not just for teenagers as menopausal acne is also a concern for some women.

A recent study by researchers at Tokyo Medical University found that drinking a glass of tomato juice a day eased symptoms. They discovered 200ml twice a day for eight weeks also helped ease cholesterol and anxiety in women. Overall, in the 93 women studied, their symptoms - including hot flushes - had almost halved

ACNE

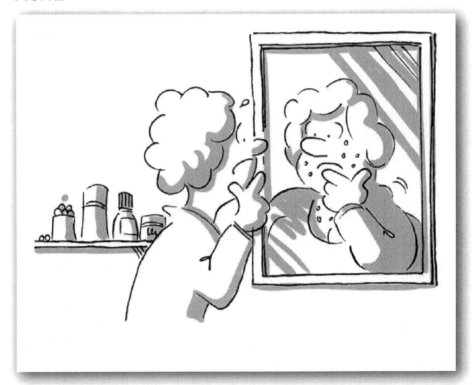

Just when you thought one of the benefits of getting older would be no more spots; acne rears its ugly head. Or heads, in the case of the worst affected.

This is because of the fluctuations in hormones which cause changes in the body's entire chemistry. Androgen levels, the male hormones in women, don't change - and this causes a stronger response to hormones such as testosterone, which stimulates sebaceous glands in the skin.

The skin then produces more sebum at the same time as cell renewal slows down, meaning blocked pores which lead to infections, pimples and other blemishes. The good news is that the reaction tends to be temporary until the body gets used to the new hormone levels.

Acne at the onset of menopause is an unpleasant surprise that many women will face. The good news that as it is generally temporary, anyone affected only needs to stay indoors for around six to nine months or invest in a mask!

VAGINAL ATROPHY

There are complaints made of vaginal dryness and painful sex because of a lack of lubrication.

The term for painful intercourse is dyspareunia, which is mostly caused by a horrendous-sounding symptom -vaginal atrophy. This means the shrinking – and eventually the death -of cells in the reproductive organs. The genitals become less elastic and the skin thinner, which leads to soreness and even inflammation.

Although the term 'atrophy' relates to more extreme symptoms such as irritation, bleeding and discharge – the very description is enough to think our lower bits are crumbling like the cliffs of Dover, with no possible chance of recovery. It's no wonder that sufferers would prefer to avoid sex altogether – no don't with the worry that bits of them could fall off at highly inappropriate points.

Joking aside, many women experience changes in the vagina and bladder as a consequence of oestrogen deficiency. This might involve changes in the structure, blood supply, support, elasticity, sensitivity, lubrication and responsiveness of the vagina.

If just treating the vagina and/or bladder symptoms of the menopause, vaginal oestrogen in the form of a very small tablet inserted with an applicator, vaginal cream, a pessary, or a vaginal ring can be used.

What is also important is to discuss the matter with your partner and, if necessary a doctor. Then you can decide what treatment is likely to suit best, depending on the symptoms and whether or not you also have bladder problems.

DIZZY SPELLS

Feeling suddenly giddy or light-headed can be alarming, but yet again this can be a sign of low oestrogen because the hormone affects our nervous system, circulation and temperature control.

When you think back to all those historic dramas when ladies were taken to faint – the youngest would be expected to be pregnant and the older ones, just old. Little did they know it was a natural adjustment in the passage of a woman through the many tribulations of life thrown upon her by hormones.

HEART PALPITATIONS

It is very common for women going through the menopause to believe they have a heart condition – a fear brought about by very noticeable palpitations – when the heart feels like it is pounding, fluttering or beating out of time.

Thankfully the symptoms are generally harmless although they should be checked out by a GP – while (guess what!) stress, alcohol, smoking, and even spicy foods can trigger them.

MEMORY LOSS

Yes, it is all perfectly normal. All that stuff when we go into another room and can't for the life of us remember why.

Dr Miriam Weber, a neuropsychologist at the University of Rochester Medical Centre, carried out a study to prove that memory loss can be a sign of the menopause – something she said would strike a chord with millions of women.

Her report confirmed that memory difficulties are one of the most common symptoms for peri-menopausal women and she added that the study suggests that, not only do the problems exist, but they become more prevalent in the first year after their last period.

The study showed what happened after 117 women were given a series of tests to do with different types of their memory. They replicated daily tasks such as learning a shopping list or series of numbers.

Researchers discovered that women in the early stage of post-menopause performed worse on measures of verbal learning, verbal memory and fine motor skills than women just before going through the menopause or two years into it. They also found symptoms such as sleep difficulties, depression and anxiety did not predict memory problems.

Dr Weber said: 'While absolute hormone levels could not be linked with cognitive function, it is possible that the fluctuations that occur during this time could play a role in the memory problems that many women experience. Parts of the brain most dependent on oestrogen, which diminishes during the menopause, are important for verbal memory and processing speed.'

Two years ago, at the age of 47, my friend Mandy noticed her short-term memory wasn't as good as it used to be. It happened at the same time as she noticed she was becoming more emotional.

'I'd go to the shop for some bread but buy everything else apart from what I went into the shop for. I can be thinking of doing one thing and the next second have completely forgotten what it is, which can make me feel like I'm going mad.'

She added that on one occasion she got into her car to go and pick her husband up from the station and completely forgot where she was going.

'I was driving around for fifteen minutes trying to remember what I had to do. It felt like my brain had completely shut down,' added Mandy.

Dr Weber said the most important thing that women need to be reassured of is that these problems, while frustrating, are normal and, in all likelihood, temporary.

Dr John Stevenson, a menopause expert based at Royal Brompton Hospital in London, said: 'When women discover it's probably a symptom of the menopause, they are usually very relieved as they feared they might be suffering from Alzheimer's disease.'

❖ *Mood changes can trigger the release of histamine, responsible for inflammatory response, causing itchy skin. You may blush more easily, too*

SMOKERS SUFFER MORE

Women who report the worst symptoms, according to a number of studies, are more likely to be smokers – and/or overweight.

Researcher, BjørnGjelsvik from the University of Oslo, found that women in a Norwegian study who had more problems with symptoms were also more likely to be daily smokers, have lower educational levels and were not living with a partner.

"We controlled for economic status, but we did not find any differences there. Nor did we find any correlation between obesity and problematic symptoms, or between a lack of physical activity and symptoms," Gjelsvik said.

Gjelsvik believes that smoking is the only well-documented lifestyle factor that clearly makes menopause more difficult for women.

"Women who smoke experience menopause earlier and more dramatically than women who do not," he said.

PSYCHIATRIC DISORDERS

There is now proof that the menopause can actually drive you mad.

According to psychiatrist and UCLA anxiety expert, Jason Eric Schiffman, there is an absolute connection between hormonal changes and psychiatric symptoms in general, and women can have increased risk for psychiatric disorders during the change.

He said: 'Women in the peri-menopausal period are more likely to experience panic attacks and other anxiety symptoms than other women of the same age who are either pre- or postmenopausal.'

But the madness isn't permanent. Mr Schiffman reassuringly tells us that once menopause passes, many women find that their level of anxiety decreases.

CRAWLING SKIN

Many women have been known to repeatedly check their cats for fleas, or insist on an insect infestation – thanks to another lesser known symptom of the menopause: crawling skin.

It is described as a sensation of ants crawling over your skin, or even under it, and is brought about by the skin receptors adapting to having less oestrogen than it's been used to.

The sensation is more annoying that harmful and can start at any time before the menopause, lasting periodically until it has completely gone. Called formication (yes, with an 'm'), it is also liked to other skin symptoms such as general itching – caused by skin getting thinner and dryer – and also pins and needles.

ACHING JOINTS

Bending down to scratch the itchy bits can become a problem in the menopausal years too. Creaking knees, aching backs and a lack of flexibility are yet more possible side effects from the departure of Mrs Oestrogen.

Dr Rod Hughes, consultant rheumatologist at St Peter's Hospital, Chertsey, Surrey, said that menopausal women tend to get soreness at the base of the thumbs, the elbows, knees, back and neck.

As if that wasn't enough, he added that hip pain can also be a problem, in particular over the outside of the hips.

Many women think this is to do with the hip joints themselves and start worrying about major surgery for replacements.

But these aches have nothing to do with the actual joints, which still move freely. He explains that the aches are brought about by tenderness in tissues between muscles – and again down to falling levels of oestrogen and subsequent inflammation in the soft tissues.

He believes that stretching exercises – such as yoga and Pilates – can help, as can losing weight and building more muscle (with weight training).

Again, the symptoms are likely to be temporary. So no signing up for that stair lift just yet.

Sex and the Shitty

Anyone who has seen Sex In The City might feel the world is on fire with raging lust and constant desire, which is fine if all your 'bits' are in working order.

For those of us who have contemplated a lifetime commitment to any available convent, as long as it gets us out of bedroom duty, it can all seem very out of sync with reality.

Sex is routinely cited as a key factor for a happy and healthy relationship. It's one of those things that might always have had something of an imbalance but is generally around in sufficient supply to keep both sides of a partnership happy.

That's until the Big M kicks in and women largely lose interest in anything physical, particularly if it requires any effort or enthusiasm.

While there is a clearly defined physical response to arousal, there is also a large psychological component. Losing interest in sex in the menopause has traditionally been seen as normal.

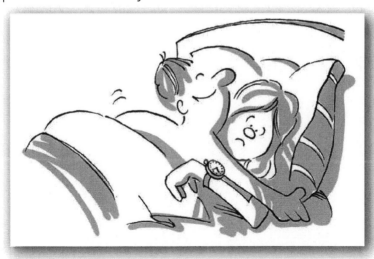

My friend, Carol, was horrified when her mother in law said she gave up all physical relations with her husband at the age of 54.

'She told me she couldn't be bothered, and as she also had a dodgy hip used that as her excuse to remain celibate for the rest of their marriage, which ended on his death. The poor man went nearly thirty years without intercourse – well, as far as we know.'

Women might attribute the lack of libido to the strain within the relationship or familiarity with their partner—being bored. They feel like they can take it or leave it, and unless their partner is pushing them, they may hope for a quiet night rather than an early night.

But does that mean we are ignoring the possibility that our relationships, while changing, could get a darn sight better?

The same friend said she hadn't understood her mother in law until she hit fifty and realised that there is a whole world that hasn't been spoken about.

'What she was really saying is that the life had been drained from her. She just couldn't be bothered during the menopause and, once the rot set in, sex was a taboo.'

Anna's mother in law may well have been able to learn how to take advantage of a new era in her life but those few years kicked her libido into touch, where it lay on the touchline – ignored and irrelevant.

Of course it isn't just the fact that the desire is missing. Many women start to encounter pain instead of pleasure during sex – robbing us of the chance to achieve orgasm and therefore have an incentive to take part.

A number of online surveys, where women can respond anonymously to questions about sensitive subjects showed that over half of the 1002 respondents of one survey reported vaginal discomfort.

Although the vast majority – nearly 90 per cent - felt that an active sex life was important to their relationship, only 20% had discussed their symptoms with a healthcare professional, 61% hid their symptoms from their partner, 60% felt less confident as a result of their symptoms and 42% made excuses not to have sex because of the discomfort.

They didn't use the real reason, though, preferring instead to say they were too tired, had a headache or not in the mood.

But all is not lost. The magnetic therapy provided a great help in this area for me but there are also many lubricants readily available that will provide the moisture the vagina needs. It is best to use those meant for the purpose – rather than any passing oils, foodstuffs or chocolate-based spreads – on the basis they are sterile and therefore discourage bacterial growth.

However should an urge come along and you don't want to waste it – after all, it could be a while before the next one – then there's no harm in trying out coconut, olive or even baby oil. Just test them out first in case they do irritate and add insult to atrophy.

TAKE YOUR TIME

Another opportunity not to be missed is the demand for extended foreplay. During parenthood or busy schedules 'the quickie' might have been the answer at the time (and still could be if it is a case of getting through the process before going off the idea completely) but older ladies need more time.

Rushing into the main act might mean there's not enough moisture so make sure your partner takes time and puts in the effort. If you're up for it, that's also the time to talk about fantasies or doing something different – it could be just what you need to spice up the whole sorry business of sex.

Unlike Carol's mother in law, many menopausal women say you have to 'use it or lose it' and so it could make sense to 'fake it until you make it'.

Having more and frequent sex can improve the blood flow of the organs, improve their elasticity and prevent dryness.

> ❖ *A tip regarding more frequent sex: If penetration or other sex acts brings too much pain, there's no reason why you have to involve a partner. A good way of getting back in touch with yourself is... to get back in touch with yourself. Alone.*

If the tried and trusted methods aren't working there are a number of natural products claiming to help women regain their sexual desire.

These include things such as Sarsaparilla and Tribulus, alongside various proteins and flavonoids that improve libido by stimulating sex hormones directly through the brain.

Damiana is a shrub that has been used as an aphrodisiac even by the old Mayan tribes. It is native in south-western parts of Mexico, Central America and the Caribbean. It is produces a mild sedative effect, which then increases the desire for intimacy and intensifies desire.

The inappropriately named chaste berry is native to Mediterranean areas which is claimed to help balance hormones and increase libido by heightening sensitivity an also stimulating natural lubrication.

Of course if after all this you still think your partner is about as attractive as a warthog with acne, then it might be worth some couples counselling.

Open dialogue with your partner, guided by a therapist, can bring up any issues that might be contributing to the problem, such as stress within the relationship, self-image problems and lack of communication. A trained sex therapist can help bring these matters to the surface so they don't escalate into a major problem.

There's no quick fix for loss of sex drive for women – as yet nothing to really equate to the male sex enhancer, Viagra - but there are things that can help.

First and foremost is speaking honestly with your partner about your feelings.

Maybe not all of them because he may not want to hear that you're bored with the same old routines and can't be bothered to chase the long-lost-lust unless it's in preparation for a night with Michael Buble…

❖ *I see menopause as the start of the next fabulous phase of life as a woman. Now is a time to 'tune in' to our bodies and embrace this new chapter in our lives. If anything, I feel more myself and love my body more now, at 58 years old, than ever before. – Kim Cattrall*

Despite all the horror stories, suggesting your nether regions will turn into prune-like relics of a forgotten youth, there is plenty to suggest that a decent sex life will resume.

Perhaps only a man such as Irwin Goldstein, MD, the director of San Diego Sexual Medicine at Alvarado Hospital, would suggest you can have the greatest sex life on earth, but it's true that the problems of the old 'monthlies' interrupting coitus have gone. If the kids are grown up and the nest is truly empty, then you can have sex in any room in the house – whenever you like.

Mind you, according to evolutionary geneticists from Canada's McMaster University, it is men's drive for sex – and their tendency to choose younger mates – that leads women to menopause in first place.

Although there has been some thought that the menopause exists so that older women don't reproduce so they can care for younger women's children – such as their grandchildren – a researcher from Oxford University added to the argument that it is men's fault that the menopause exists.

Dr Maxwell Burton-Chellew said he thinks it is the human male preference for younger females and the lack of reproduction that has given rise to menopause.

Using computer modelling, the team from McMaster's concluded "preferential mating" was the evolutionary answer - men of all ages choosing younger women as partners, which meant there was "no purpose" in older women continuing to be fertile.

Prof Rama Singh, an evolutionary geneticist who led the study, said men choosing younger mates were "stacking the odds" against continued fertility.

He told the BBC: "There is evidence in human history; there was always a preference for younger women."

However, Prof Singh stressed they were looking at human development many thousands of years ago - rather than current social patterns, so before we go and start beating up any partner who might cast an eye in a downward age direction – the trend could reverse.

Extended longevity, plus later childbirth, could eventually alter the timing of the menopause – even if it is in generations to come.

"The social system is changing. There are women who are starting families later, because of education or a career."

He suggested this trend would mean those women would have a later menopause, and those genes would be passed on to their daughters "with the possibility of menopausal age being delayed".

Regardless of what researchers may say, evidence suggests that older women – with those partners who aren't seeking a younger woman – are enjoying sex in their later years, more so than their parents and grandparents.

It is quite possible that stresses of work, career and money have lessened and there's more time for evenings out or just to relax.

'Time is a huge factor,' says Amanda Richards, MD, an associate professor of obstetrics and gynaecology at the University of Miami's Miller School of Medicine.

'Menopause is a very defining time for most women, many of whom realise that they have put their sexuality on the back burner for way too long, and if they don't use it, they will lose it for good,' she said.

Margaret E. Wierman, MD, a professor of medicine, physiology, and biophysics at the University of Colorado Health Sciences Centre, in Denver, said: 'There's some data to suggest that women become less inhibited as they age, so it's often a time of relaxation and being comfortable with who you are, and that often improves sexual functioning and sexual performance,'

So maybe vaginal atrophy, waning desire and a general lack of interest in sex are only minor stumbling blocks in the progress of a woman from one era to another – and for those who think they'll never want to share an 'early night' again, hold on.. the new you could be just around the corner.

❖ *US superstar Whoopi Goldberg, 58, has never been one to hold back about anything. And in 2012, she confessed to experiencing menopausal symptoms on-air during a political discussion on talk show 'The View'. 'You know what?' she commented. 'I just had a big ol' hot flush. And my underwear is wet. So I have to go.' Whoopi has also talked openly about the fluctuations in her sex drive: 'One minute I'm like, "Yeah! I can't wait for it." The next I'm saying, "Oh, God, go away."'*

The Male Menopause

While much has been made of how women change in older life, there's mounting evidence to suggest that men have their own type of mid-life crisis.

Not just the type that gives them personal permission to buy a motorbike, unsuitable underpants and grow a ponytail, but a genuine hormone-related, debilitating kind of trauma that could have a dramatic effect on quality of life.

The symptoms aren't necessarily the same. If men suddenly gained weight around the middle, lacked energy, were irritable and lacked virility we'd either be accusing them of a hangover – or an affair – rather than worrying about the natural signs of aging.

However, according to various reports there are an increasing number of men who are suffering from their own hormonal imbalances, most of which are going undiagnosed and untreated.

Known as Testosterone Deficiency Syndrome, or Andropause, it is still relatively unrecognised in the UK although more official bodies are popping up to at least talk about it, if not treat it. For example the Andropause Society has undertaken considerable research and offer some hope for men who want to improve their hormone levels.

The advice isn't dissimilar to that given to women – moderate alcohol intake, reduce stress and generally follow a healthier lifestyle. According to the Society, if a man is diagnosed as being testosterone deficient then these measures should be adopted alongside any treatment prescribed to assist a man to return his hormone levels to what is deemed the normal range.

Regardless of diagnose, a recent Angus Reid survey found that 70% of the general public share the belief that men experience a mid-life stage similar to women's menopause.

However, whether the term 'male menopause' is accurate is a debatable point among medics such as Dr Geoffrey Hackett, sexual health specialist at Good Hope Hospital in Birmingham, and the former chair of the British Society for Sexual Medicine.

'Only twenty per cent of males experience low levels of testosterone whereas all women go through the menopause,' he said.

However he does believe that male hormone replacement therapy is valid and worthwhile particularly when treating libido and erectile issues – citing it as both safe and effective.

This view may give reason to why the more medical term of 'Andropause' isn't categorised as dramatically as it is in women – there are no periods to stop or obvious physical changes – but a more gradual decline in mood and energy as well as a lower libido and lack of physical agility.

There are also more serious health risks implied as the drop in testosterone can also contribute to problems such as heart disease and weak bones.

At about the time I was evaluating my life as a woman, my husband confessed to having a similarly cathartic experience regarding his age.

Although he couldn't list quite the same physical symptoms, his mid-life event happened when he was taking stock of his achievements and evaluating his life. He woke up to the fact he was 50, not so much in crisis mode, by facing a crossroads. It was time to take stock, and take advantage of a new era.

We'd been through quite a lot, particularly looking after our parents, and when that stopped we both looked back – and then realised we had so much in front of us as well.

He said: 'Time felt like it had passed so quickly. As a young man you look forward and plan then suddenly you turn fifty and you wonder where it's all gone.'

The feeling was a surprise but not uncomfortable. While Joe said that time did seem to have passed very quickly, his hopes for another thirty good years of life propelled him into a new era.

'It was time to Fight Back at 50. I did a lot of things I'd been meaning to, started to take my health seriously and looked at what I wanted to do. It was time to take life on at full speed.'

One of the possible reasons that the Andropause hasn't been routinely diagnosed over the years could be that men just won't admit they don't feel as young as they used to. It is bad enough to get many of them to admit any health problem at all – but one that affects their sex drive?

As with women's menopause, doctors won't always look at low testosterone levels as the culprit behind symptoms either – with many middle aged men being diagnosed with depression.

Just like when my doctor suggested I buy bigger pants, doctors dealing with male issues of mid-life might just tell their patients they are 'no longer spring chickens' and they should expect their foot to come off the pedal a bit.

Maybe that is why so many men in their fifties go and buy fast cars or find young women. Being told you're losing your essential power, or just feeling it, can cause a huge psychological issue.

However, there are new blood testing methods available which, alongside increased interest in men's aging among medical researchers, could soon make a difference. Which is good news for those ladies, who, struggling to find the key to their own libido have realised they're barking up the wrong tree – because their husband is as knackered as they are.

Again the comparisons to the women's menopause have to be made because not all men will suffer although a decline in testosterone levels will occur in virtually all men.

Medical journals have been discussing this for decades at it is only the availability of a hormone test for men, more recently, that has given the study more impetus.

Until that point, conventional medicine denied there was such a thing as male menopause or Andropause. Yet physiology and endocrinology text- books as far back as the 1920's address the lowering of testosterone in late middle age as the male 'point of no return'.

One reason that it might not have been looked into in any greater detail for such a long time was the fact that testosterone was a dirty word.

It was blamed for everything from cancer to causing war, criminal behaviour and rape. It is easy to see why many doctors would be reluctant to suggest prescribing testosterone just to make men feel a bit better about themselves.

As a woman's ovaries pack up in mid-life, a man's testicles stop making testosterone and progesterone – the latter hormone being needed to keep testosterone from turning into oestrogen - while their adrenals and body fat keep making oestrogen.

The potential overload of oestrogen, particularly with the amount that is now in the environment through our water supplies and other sources, means that men going through the Andropause can expect:

- Lack of morning erections when awaking – because of the fact testosterone is no longer being produced at night.
- The penis is also likely to shrink and have weaker and less frequent erections
- There will be increased hair growth on the back but loss of hair from the head
- More fat around the breast area – or 'moobs'
- Loss of muscle mass, flabbiness and loose skin
- Loss of 'get up and go'
- Lowered or lack of libido

- Smaller less pleasurable orgasms
- Back pains,
- Generalized weakness,
- Swollen prostate.

As if that wasn't enough, bits of the brain that are responsible for the 'happiness' drug in our system – Dopamine – start to die off. This is the true source of desire and low levels can induce a lack of interest in sex.

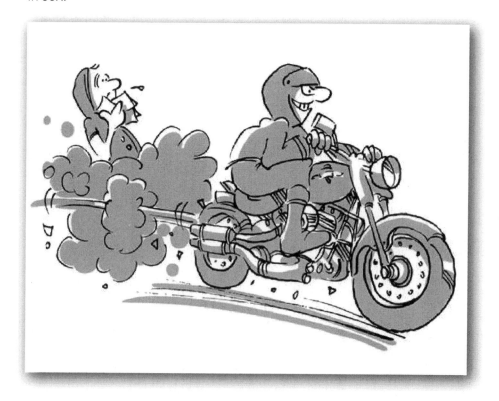

'Oh, I can get Viagra' might be the common response to such a litany of horrors but some of these things can't be fixed with a little blue pill.

❖ *Male menopause is a lot more fun than female menopause. With female menopause you gain weight and get hot flashes. Male menopause you get to date young girls and drive motorcycles. John Wayne.*

Any male who has signs of low testosterone should talk to their doctor – not least because many of these symptoms can be caused by diseases that can be dangerous and should be ruled out. These days' testosterone levels are checked with a simple blood test – although normal levels are different for each man so it might be difficult to get an accurate diagnosis.

If low testosterone is diagnosed, it is worth thinking about visiting a specialist, such as an endocrinologist or urologist, who can discuss possible treatments.

Mel Gibson famously suffered from some kind of mid-life crisis in 2008 which could be attributed to the symptoms of Andropause.

He said in a letter: 'I need to do something - something lasting, not just a band aid."

He'd gone on to say he didn't know why he was so 'whacky and depressed' but that he needed to get well and 're-enter life'

Mel referred to his holistic doctor and claimed that he was going through some kind of male menopause.

'This isn't who I was meant to be - I know it!"

❖ *The male equivalent of HRT - male hormone replacement treatment is gaining ground among men and, over the past decade, prescriptions for testosterone gels and injections have doubled, to 300,000 a year.*

Although weight gain, lack of energy and poor concentration can be a sign of low hormone levels it isn't always going to be the case.

If the man in your life is smoking, eating kebabs and curries most nights and drinking his weight in lager while refusing to do anything more energetic than go to the loo on a slightly more regular basis than normal, then it could just be lifestyle.

In America, where drug companies can advertise directly to the public, men spend nearly £2.5 billion a year on testosterone - but this is despite the lack of data on its long-term safety, and the fact that symptoms don't always improve, according to the consultant endocrinologist at the Royal Victoria Hospital in Newcastle upon Tyne, Dr Richard Quinton.

He has seen many cases of the male menopause and older men with low testosterone – both he believes are the 'normal symptoms of unhealthy ageing'. Professor Fred Wu, director of the Andrology Research Unit in Manchester, has a similar opinion. According to recent reports, he believes that many cases of symptoms associated with low testosterone are more to do with men who haven't been looking after themselves.

'These are normal symptoms of unhealthy ageing,' he said. 'Obese men with low testosterone normally find their levels bounce back when they lose weight or get control of their diabetes.'

❖ *Losing weight is the single most effective lifestyle change for boosting testosterone levels. A man who sheds ten per cent of his weight — shown to be achievable with regular exercise, a healthy diet and cutting down on alcohol — raises testosterone levels substantially, according to the European Male Ageing Study in 2013.*

Depression and excessive drinking have an impact according to Professor Gary Wittert, head of medicine at the University of Adelaide, Australia, who also think that changes in physical and mental health are more commonly down to lifestyle.

Work and family problems – such as a menopausal partner – can also contribute and this is sometimes where the 'talking therapies' such as counselling can help. It's often difficult enough to get any man along to such sessions, let alone one with hormone issues, so it might be a case of finding other coping strategies.

It can be particularly hard to cope with your partner's 'menopausal' symptoms if you're experience similar - or worse - problems yourself.

Personal development specialist Jane C Woods offers these tips: 'Remember the advice from airline safety demonstrations about putting your own oxygen mask on before helping anyone else? It will be hard to be understanding towards your partner is you don't feel good yourself, so set him a positive example by showing you care about your health and seeking help for any symptoms you have. And try to show some empathy. Your partner may have trouble identifying what ails him as being part of a natural process, so he may choose to ignore it. The best thing you can do for him - and you - is to take his symptoms seriously and listen.

Celebrity Menopause

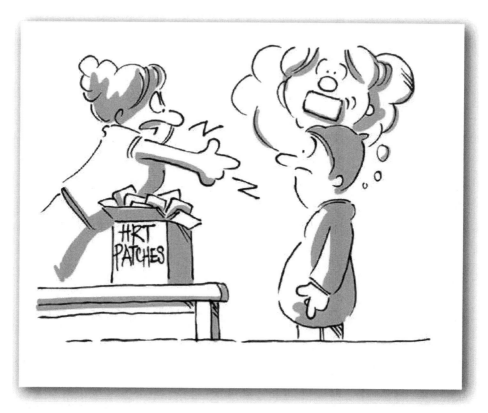

It doesn't matter who you are, what you earn or how many people know your name – if your hormones are going to play hide and seek, you can easily get caught out.

Rosemary Conley, the woman behind the diet and fitness classes of the same name, started taking HRT in her early 50s and said it was one of the best decisions she ever made.

'Before I started going through the menopause I was convinced it wouldn't affect me. I was fit, ate healthily and had an extremely positive outlook so I presumed I was mentally and physically equipped to deal with it. I was wrong - like most women, my menopausal symptoms really started to affect my life. I became tired, lethargic and miserable. '

She said she felt like she was firing on two cylinders and so went to her doctor to enquire about HRT.

'He did warn me there was a minute risk of developing breast cancer but I felt that the benefits - a normal happy lifestyle - outweighed the dangers. HRT has had a really good effect on my life. Not only is it helping lower my risk of heart disease, it is also maintaining the health of my bones which lowers my chances of developing osteoporosis. '

Surprisingly she also said that she weighed less than before she started treatment, without changing her diet or exercise regime.

'Before my menopause I really felt my age. But now I've recaptured the energy I had in my youth and feel 20 again,' she said.

Fleetwood Mac singer, Stevie Nicks, has spoken about her difficult menopause and how she has dealt with the symptoms.

She said that getting on stage is fine – it's getting off that's the problem.

'When you're on stage you have to forget about it. There is no dizzies, there is no cramps, there is no menopause. All there is, is the audience and what you do. So you feel great for those two hours. And when I come off stage, then I can burst into tears.

Linda Barker says the menopause hit her "like a freight train" – but a change of lifestyle gave her a new energy.

In an interview with the Daily Express, she said: 'Brain fog descended as I became forgetful and emotional – at the age of 48 I just wasn't feeling in control of my life, which wasn't like me at all.

She said her biggest problem was anxiety, which would come on after a hot flush – and everything would take on monumental proportions.

Linda added that the change is an appropriate name for it all because everything shifts. 'Your physical being, your mental approach, the way you look.'

She took HRT for a while but after speaking to a GP believed she was only delaying the inevitable and so changed to a natural approach – adopting a diet based on soya beans and oats. She also took black cohosh while focusing on load-bearing exercise at the gym to ward off osteoporosis.

Talking about her appearance on the TV show, Splash, where she took part in a diving contest, she said she wouldn't have had the courage to take part when she was younger.

'I think that's hormonal – you get a bit more testosterone after the menopause.'

Unlike some women who feel their career could be jeopardised by age, she thinks it is a bit easier for women in the entertainment business these days.

'We have amazing actresses such as Judi Dench and Helen Mirren who aren't afraid to talk about how old they are the issues they've faced, the wrinkles they've grown. We need to share those experiences. '

Gloria Hunniford, the TV and radio presenter, reportedly has a different view.

Her menopause started in her mid-forties but she said she didn't suffer much at all.

'I had no hot flushes. All that really happened is that my periods went away,' she said.

Despite pressure from her GP she declined HRT because of a family history of breast cancer and instead took lots of supplements such as the vitamins E and C and phytosome, prescribed by a homeopathic doctor.

'I also ate an exceptionally healthy diet - lots of broccoli and leafy vegetables...I did plenty of exercise, making sure I walked lots and went on my exercise bike.

Angela Rippon is reported as having a very pragmatic view towards the menopause.

She said: 'My attitude to the menopause is the same as my attitude to measles. As a child you have to have measles and as a woman in your 50s, you have to have the menopause.

When she was offered HRT she weighed up the pros and cons and decided to give it a go – and took it for five years before opting for a more natural solution.

'I decided to stop. There was no major reason. I just felt my body might benefit from something natural. I decided to take red clover instead and I feel as good as ever.'

She also believes many women can help themselves through the menopause by eating healthily and keeping fit and happy.

❖ *"After the menopause is a good time, honest! Once the flushes stop and things settle. I've got more energy and things start fitting into place emotionally." - Julie Walters*

Comedy star Jennifer Saunders was prescribed the oestrogen-blocking drug Tamoxifen as the final stage of her successful breast cancer treatment in 2009.

She told the Daily Telegraph in an interview: 'It plunges you into the menopause in one fell swoop. 'It's fairly brutal and you go through all the accompanying side effects: hot flushes; weight gain; a sense of mourning for lost youth, sexiness and somehow the point in anything'.

She sought help from a psychologist and got some medication to help lift her out of the subsequent depression.

Actress Jane Seymour began HRT soon after she first experienced menopausal symptoms at the age of 47. She stopped after seven years and, like many other women, opted for a diet high in natural phytoestrogens instead. She is also reported to have taken red clover and alfalfa supplements before switching back to HRT when her mood swings and hot flushes came back.

She said of her experience: 'Each woman has to create her own way of dealing with the menopause - one that works for her.'

Actress Patsy Kensit had an emergency hysterectomy in June 2013 after two tumours were found in her womb, which led to the onset of menopause. She had a marked response to HRT until her body got used to its effects and she said in an interview on This Morning: 'The menopause is a taboo subject that has a stigma, and people don't want to discuss it.'

❖   *"The best aspect of the menopause is that it gives a woman licence to behave badly!" - Kathy Lette*

Singer/songwriter Tori Amos has taken inspiration from her experience with the menopause, using the ageing process to spark the album, Unrepentant Geraldines.

In an interview in The Huffington Post, she said she found menopause to be a tough road and a tough teacher.

'Finding your own self-acceptance and sensuality within it is, well, sometimes it's a real hunt. You have to dive in there because of the feelings that you're having…There is a quiet, silent grieving that happens through menopause. It might happen in a way where you're not aware of it but you can begin to lose memory for a minute — you can forget things — and you're very aware that you're going through a different process, a different phase of life.'

Former Loose Women start and actress, Denise Welch, reckons the menopause was the best thing that ever happened to her – even though its onset sent her into a depression, something she'd battled all her life.

She said that she was working on the TV show, Waterloo Road, when she was trying to work through her depression but losing the battle.

Higher doses of drugs made no difference and soon Denise started to think her problems were hormonally triggered – particularly as the depression set in after the birth of her first son.

She went to see a specialist, Professor John Studd, who discovered that Denise was almost completely deficient in oestrogen.

'When he prescribed it for me, alongside the low-dose anti-depressants I was taking, everything got better. Now I think that episode of depression I had (while working on Waterloo Road) had been the start of my menopause.'

She added that if the menopause hadn't triggered another bout of depression she may never have gone to see Professor Studd, who transformed her.

"So you could say that the menopause saved my life. Incredibly, it has been the best thing that ever happened to me.

Crimes of the Menopause

While many women can blame the menopause for things they might not otherwise do – such as using their partners' toothbrush to clean the toilet or forgetting to send their Mother-in-Law a birthday card - there are a few who have managed to escape jail sentences because of their sudden lack of social concern.

Although there have been no solid studies to prove that menopausal women turn into rampaging shoplifters, folklore suggests it happens while documented incidents cite a woman's time of life for being the reason they are behaving irrationally, rather than criminally. In most cases, any such crime would be considered 'out of character'.

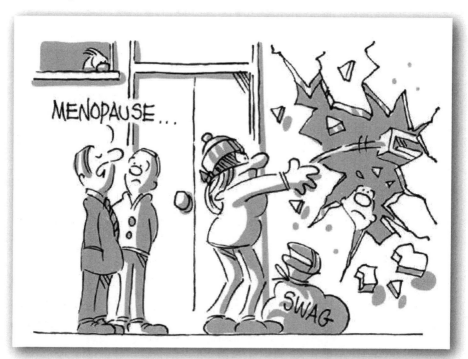

A solicitor suggested to Carlow District Court in Ireland that his client, a woman of a certain age, may have shoplifted because she was middle-aged and going through the menopause.

He was representing a woman who'd pleaded guilty to the theft of 50 Euro's worth of groceries at a local supermarket.

The lawyer said that while his client was of good character, he didn't know why she shoplifted the goods. It wasn't in her nature and went against her otherwise good, law-abiding personality. He continued that she was middle-aged and that he'd read an article linking shoplifting with menopausal women.

Judge William Harnett wasn't convinced, however, replying that theft was a serious offence that cost retailers a lot of money – and imposed a five hundred Euro fine on the woman.

Similarly, Asmita Patel was in the midst of the menopause, in 2007, when she stole almost £5,700 from elderly pensioners while working as an assistant at a post office in Kent. The only reason that could be found for her dishonesty was that she was going through the menopause.

Patel, who said she didn't know why she did it, was sentenced to 12 weeks imprisonment suspended for two years and ordered to do 240 hours unpaid work and pay £480 costs.

Judge Philip Statman said he was only just persuaded he could avoid sending Patel, who admitted four theft charges, to jail.

"When I came into court today I had in mind you would be going to prison immediately for 12 weeks," he said.

"I have thought long and hard about how the public as a whole can best be protected and would react if I were to send you to prison.

"For this type of offence is extremely serious. There are those who remind me the prisons are overcrowded and you pose no real risk.'

Well, no risk other than to those living with a menopausal thief – on the basis this was the only 'crime' of her condition.

In the USA, a former Elbert County assessor, P J Trostel, could have had the book thrown at her for her mismanagement of money and the 'hostile environment' she created at work.

Anyone living with someone on the verge of a hormone collapse can understand both those charges although in this case the sentence could have been six years in jail.

Judge Jeffrey Holmes thought about it but eventually settled for just two months in prison with probation and community service.

This was after she blamed the menopause on her 'out of character' behaviour.

Trostel was indicted by a grand jury in September 2010 on charges that included embezzlement, forgery, theft and perjury.

She was accused of using her county credit card to purchase gift cards and then buy personal items. She was also charged with purchasing two printers with public funds, which makes me wonder if it was to print out the various symptoms and possible solutions to the change of life – because that would take two printers, and a hell of a lot of ink!

In asking for leniency, Trostel and her lawyer said a variety of factors led her to make bad decisions. Those included depression, symptoms from menopause, medications and stress from family and work.

"Some of the things I don't even have an answer," she said. "I know I made terrible judgments and decisions."

I feel the woman's pain. My decisions became erratic when I hit 52. Until then I'd been capable, easy-going and even laughed at my husband's jokes. All that had stopped.

Up until the point of her criminal activity, Trostel had a clean record. She clearly gave the impression of being able to do her job. In a similar way I'd shown such capability – having given up my career in the theatre to care for my mother-in-law who fell ill with Alzheimer's. That isn't a job for someone with a short fuse or lack of energy.

In this woman's case, the court was so concerned about Trostel reacting to employees who testified against her they hired security to monitor the floor of her office – even though she signed herself off work as soon as she was charged.

No doubt she recognised her temper could take her over and turn her into the beast she was being described as.

"This type of activity is not acceptable," said the Judge. "She needs assistance that only mandatory confinement would provide."

While I'm not for a minute suggesting that all middle aged women should go around embezzling councils and hoping to get away with it, there is something to be said for offering 'mandatory confinement' as a possible solution. Preferably in a spa hotel with room service and a flat screen TV.

Not knowing the full story, or what this person was like before she was arrested, I wouldn't want to make too many assumptions but I do recognise extreme personality change in otherwise sensible females.

I have another friend who went from being very outgoing, attractive and kind – to the type of person you'd cross the road to avoid. She thought nothing of her 'honesty' in telling total strangers they were idiots (or worse) for the smallest of offences such as dropping their purse in the supermarket queue, or failing to turn right at a busy junction in what she considered to be a reasonable timescale. Her hairdresser offended her by suggesting a slightly more flattering cut for her 'fuller face' and she left the salon with wet hair and an unpaid bill for the colour and wash.

She has now become the sort of woman who would instil fear into every flight passenger should she have become a pilot.

One menopausal woman who did get a long incarceration for her crimes, despite claims of hormonal imbalance, was a former third-grade teacher who admitted to taking photos of her students dancing in their underwear. She provided a laundry list of bizarre excuses for her behaviour – the main one, of course, being her time of life.

Kimberly Crain of Oklahoma was charged with exploitation and pornography charges before claiming that the menopause, hypnosis, an 'emotionally absent' husband, coupled with depression led to her illegal acts.

Of course the husband could have been absent because of her type of Jekyll and Hyde personality exchange - and the depression could be that which comes with a new life stage. Whatever had happened hadn't been previously recorded – again because of otherwise good character.

On this occasion, and probably for very good reason, no leniency was granted, but it shows that hormonal activity can either be the reason, or be cited as the reason, for a wide variety of crimes and 'out of character' behaviour.

❖ *I'm not surprised menopausal women are caught shoplifting. I have nothing but compassion for them now I know what this is like. I have caught myself on more than one occasion heading towards the supermarket exit with a basket of strange odds and sods I had no idea I wanted and had forgotten I hadn't even paid for. Melissa Kite, Daily Mail 2014*

Benefits of the Menopause

OK, so we've talked about all the signs, symptoms and solutions of the menopause. We've brought it out in the open and given 'The Big M' permission to be talked about – usually in all its gory detail.

But is it really all bad?

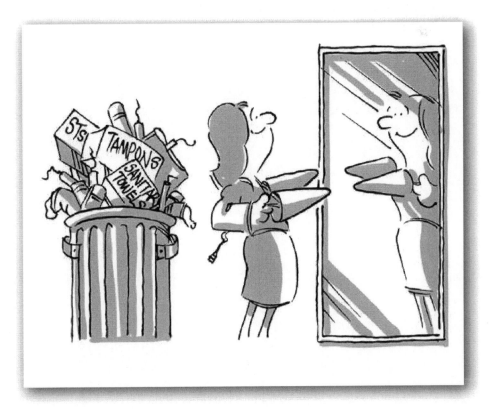

In many ways there are some great bits to no more periods. No more periods, for a start. Then there's the chance to wear white trousers without having to think what day in the cycle it is – and no more buying tampons or sanitary towels (still taxed by the Government at 5% despite being necessary items for a good number of the population).

And these days, it is not hard to find examples of successful older women – we've already mentioned the oft-hailed older beauties, Helen Mirren and Judi Dench and there are many more such as Meryl Streep and Julie Walters; but what about politicians who find true power in their later years - for example, US Secretary of State Hillary Clinton and German chancellor Angela Merkel.

In an article for Time Magazine, a psychiatrist stated that Hillary Clinton is the perfect age to be president.

The article said: 'A woman emerging from the transition of peri-menopause blossoms. It is a time for redefining and refining what it is she wants to accomplish in her third act. And it happens to be excellent timing for the job Clinton is likely to seek. Biologically speaking, postmenopausal women are ideal candidates for leadership. They are primed to handle stress well, and there is, of course, no more stressful job than the presidency.'

Perhaps politics allows women to be 'neutral' in their position as it doesn't rely on levels of sexuality as, perhaps, the entertainment industry might do.

If we take Madonna as an example, she will be 60 before her current recording contract completes – yet she is still pushing the boundaries of an industry cluttered with ambitious, attractive and talented young people. She manages to beat them all with her own brand of ageless attitude.

Not only does she still rock the music world but she has gone through the menopause with no outwardly noticeable issues and gone on to write and direct films without any desire to tone down her personality or showgirl status.

Author, Vivian Diller, Ph.D., writes in her book Face It: What Women Really Feel As Their Looks Change, that it is important for Madonna to keep her power, claiming she is the ultimate re-inventor. The latest return of Madonna, according to the book, is no different to anything she's done in the past.

'She's bringing back some of what she used to represent—and her breaking sexual boundaries has always been a part of that—but at the same time becoming something more, an icon to a generation of women who want to remain vital, creative and, yes, sexual, even as they age."

Of course change will happen and Madonna can't be the 30 year old she once was. However, by allowing her ageing to be part of her public persona then, according to Diller, she'll continue to be a role model for multiple generations of women.

Angelia Jolie has been upbeat and positive about her own journey into menopause, brought about by elective operations to remove her ovaries and fallopian tubes in an attempt to reduce the chance of getting cancer. The procedure has put her into forced menopause meaning she won't be able to have any more children and will bring some changes.

She said she feels at ease at what is to come. 'Not because I am strong but because this is part of life. It's nothing to be feared,' she has told journalists.

We can't all be Madonna, Angelina, or anyone like them who have many privileges in terms of access to support and medical advice. But for those of us just hoping to get through a menopausal day without a major breakdown or locking ourselves out of the house for the fifth time in a week, there are still many good things to remember.

For any female, it is worth noting that killer whales typically become mothers between the ages of 12 and 40, but they can live for more than 90 years.

However, the males of the species only seem to make it to around the age of 50 – so maybe, evolutionary speaking, menopause serves a purpose for females of all kinds.

A report in the journal Current Biology suggests that older whales are natural, wise, leaders - while menopausal whales can guide younger members of their pod towards all the best spots for finding food such as salmon.

According to Lauren Brent of the University of Exeter, the lead author of the report, said their study is the first to demonstrate that the value gained from the wisdom of elders may be one reason female killer whales continue to live long after they have stopped reproducing.

She observed over 100 killer whales in the wild, taking into account birth and death rates as well as genetic and social information.

"In humans, it has been suggested that menopause is simply an artefact of modern medicine and improved living conditions," explained Darren Croft of the University of Exeter, the study's senior author. "However, mounting evidence suggests that menopause in humans is adaptive. In hunter-gatherers, one way that menopausal women help their relatives, and thus increase the transmission of their own genes, is by sharing food. Menopausal women may have also shared another key commodity: information."

Just as we can't all be fabulous post-menopausal celebrities, we can't all be whales either – although the study does suggest there is hope for all of us in terms of our use in later years.

Regardless of how we see the future, in terms of the here and now one of the biggest benefits to remember about the issues surrounding the menopause, such as hot flushes, tiredness, anxiety, etc., is that they tend to be temporary. They are just the body's way of dealing with changes and while irritating are rarely life-threatening.

It is also a time when many women decide to re-evaluate what isn't working in their lives. This can be routines, relationships and negativity.

American anthropologist Margaret Mead called it "menopausal zest" — an energy that women feel after the menopause which enables them to take stock of their lives.

Many decide to take a fresh look at their relationships, their professions, the ways they're caring for their own health, and the ways they want to expend their energy. It is a time to ask whether we are headed in the right direction – professionally and personally – and whether the way we're spending our time is meaningful to us.

Actress Emma Thompson had a similar pragmatism when giving an acceptance speech during an exceptionally cold night in New York.

She said: 'It's such a cold night and it's the only time I've actively been grateful for menopause. I've been entirely comfortable'

For some, the menopause brings some delightful benefits. In the case of Helena Bonham Carter, for example, the actress suggested in a recent interview that she did not have big breasts until she was going through the change.

❖   *"Old age isn't so bad when you consider the alternative."*
     ~Maurice Chevalier, New York Times, 9 October 1960

In a similar interview carried by Female First magazine the singer Sinead O'Connor claimed she was excited to be reaching menopause and looking forward to her first hot flush.

It might be easy to think about the change and the problems it can bring but women have been having problems with menstruation since time began. Individually we've all been aware of some elements such as Pre-Menstrual Syndrome (PMS) – which is very common.

Menopause says goodbye to those symptoms which, according to various experts, affect at least 85 per cent of women of child-bearing age. Being able to finally shut the door on the physical and emotional issues – from breast tenderness to food cravings and irritability – can be something of a rite of passage.

For those women who have managed to salvage anything resembling a libido, enjoyment of sex without risk of pregnancy is a huge benefit – and often cited as one of the biggest benefits of the menopause. There are also many women claiming that the levels of sexual excitement are heightened after the change – possibly due to this factor, but also down to increased confidence and knowing exactly what they want.

On a purely physical level, any woman who has suffered from fibroids – benign growths in the womb – will be pleased to know they usually stop growing or shrink during the menopause.

They tend to develop when oestrogen levels in the body are high and can be painful as well as be responsible for heavy menstrual bleeding as well as pressure on the bladder. The drop in oestrogen takes away their 'life blood' and this can be a huge relief to sufferers.

It is not uncommon for postmenopausal women to report feeling empowered, partly because of the biological changes that take place in menopause and partly because of the age at which is usually happens.

Women have been through a fair amount by this stage – pregnancy, children leaving home, careers and personal ups and downs. Many decide it is time to think how the future will shape up – not for anyone else but for just us.

Not only that, there is something bonding about sharing menopausal experiences with other women at the same stage. You can strip off your clothing together while everyone else huddles by the fire, talk to each other at 3am when for some unexplained reason you're all wide awake – and generally bemoan the lot of the female race while simultaneously rejoicing in the fact that you can throw your tampons and 'period pants' firmly in the bin.

After all, we've got through a good chunk of life and are still here to tell the tale. More's the point; there is plenty of life to come – but this time without the trials and tribulations of hormonal influence.

It's time to start the party!

Help, Information and Advice

CONTENTS

Addendum: Helpful websites and addresses

Disclaimer

The following information has been put together as a general guide as to what is available to help deal with the menopause, whether it is traditional medicine, drugs, alternative therapies or lifestyle changes.

None of the information given here is offered on a professional basis, but purely as a pointer to get advice from a registered GP or health practitioner.

A number of resources have been used to gather the information in this section and not all have been verified. Also, not all treatments are suitable for all people and it is essential that personal conditions and circumstances are considered before taking any medication or therapy.

Should you wish to consider treatment for menopausal symptoms it is recommended you do so only after suitable consultation.

The Author's Story Sheila Wenborne

When the menopause first reared its head I thought a mystery illness had taken over my body. I groaned with pain getting out of bed, I was short-tempered, emotional, suffered constant headaches and ached all over.

I'd always been active and healthy, running a successful theatre business with my husband, Joe, but when I started feeling low I put it down to the fact we'd sold the business so I could concentrate on looking after my mother in law, who'd developed Alzheimer's.

Because my moods were so erratic I thought I had depression – I'd fly into a rage if I tripped over our dog - and losing the remote control would have me in floods of tears.

I'd even put on weight for no apparent reason and was struggling to get out of bed some days.

When I went to see my GP her diagnosis was immediate, it was the menopause.

I was shocked but at 52 I had to accept that my childbearing years were over. Joe was pleased to have a diagnosis – my moods had become so bad he considered wearing a tin hat while I was around. Not only that I'd gone off any suggestion of any action in the bedroom department and was as snappy as a crocodile.

It would be easy to think there was going to be a remedy but all the first GP suggested was that I bought some bigger knickers for my expanding waistline and bought a book on the change of life.

I was horrified. What sort of advice was that? After thinking about the situation for a little longer I went back to the doctor's surgery for a second opinion and the (different) GP offered hormone replacement therapy (HRT).

I dutifully went and collected the hormone patches and as soon as I stuck them on my tummy I felt old. Apart from acting as a constant reminder of the fact I was 'old' I puffed up like a balloon and although I was in a better mood I was worried about the risks of cancer. I'd had a cervical cancer scare in my twenties and taking HRT didn't sit well with me. It really felt like I was playing Russian roulette with my life.

After a few agitated months, feeling HRT couldn't be my only option I had a light bulb moment. When our border collie suffered from arthritis we bought a magnetic collar and it seemed to work.

I'd been putting up with symptoms that didn't seem to be alleviated and so I wondered if magnetic therapy might do the same for the menopause.

I bought a clip on magnet to wear inside my knickers and within two weeks I felt better. My bloating had subsided, my mood swings had gone and I was laughing at Joe's jokes again. Surely a miracle cure!

The only thing I didn't like about the magnet was it wasn't very attractive and would sometimes show under my clothes.

I heard about a German company that made jewellery with magnets in them and within a few weeks of conducting some research had decided to set up a business selling magnetic jewellery in the UK.

I've sold hundreds of pieces that help with a range of symptoms and I would like to think that as part of that, many women have been relieved of the ravages of the menopause.

Although there is no consensus on how magnets work, it is thought that they stimulate circulation and increase endorphin levels.

A study at the University of Virginia found that magnets can reduce swelling by 50% and can also reduce muscle tension and bring oxygen and nutrients to affected areas to ease pain and speed up healing.

There will always be people who don't believe they can work and that is fine. I just want to make other women aware there is a drug-free, side-effect-free option that they might want to try if they don't like taking hormones.

I would also like other people who are suffering through the menopause, to experience the life-changing help and inspiration I've had in recent years.

This part of my life has been very much a change, but not just in the hormonal way. Since I discovered the magnets I can't believe how positive my life has become.

I was never one for the limelight but coming out of the darkness into a world full of a new kind of energy has spurred my ambition and made me realise there is so much I can do – I'd got caught up thinking about what I couldn't do any more.

The realisation was like a bolt of lightning and very soon after 'waking up' to my life, I started my own company selling the magnetic therapy products.

From someone who kept themselves to themselves I became something of an overnight success, with articles written about my story in the Sunday Mirror, The Daily Mail, Woman magazine and various other publications.

My business, Aura[3], is becoming a household name as I am thrust directly into the public eye. I'm loving the new me, the person who is looking to expand their own range of products while finding new ways to help people who are experiencing problems with not just the menopause but also the general niggles of reaching middle age.

Extra laughter lines come with extra laughter and need to be celebrated. Mature skin has its issues but also has its triumphs and in recognition of that I am developing a natural, organic skincare range. I'm also looking at many other ways to assist people in their transition into a different phase of their life – a life that should be positive, purposeful and happy.

There is so much that can be done and so much to achieve that the train isn't going to stop at magnets!

The menopause started as one of the most terrifying times in my life but it's allowed me to become the real me. It's the single most positive time I've been able to define in my life; it's certainly not the end..... for me it's just the beginning and it can be for you too.

You can find out more about me, Sheila Wenborne and Aura[3] products by visiting
www.aura3.co.uk
Or follow Aura[3] on Facebook and Twitter
Facebook: Aura3uk
Twitter: @aura3uk

Or you can follow me personally via
www.sheilawenborne.com
Facebook: SheilaWenborne
Twitter: @sheilawenborne

Other Options
HRT – Hormone Replacement Therapy

According to the NHS Choices, hormone replacement therapy (HRT) is a treatment used to relieve symptoms of the menopause. It replaces those female hormones that are starting to wane.

Oestrogen and progesterone play important roles in a woman's body and it is well established that falling levels can cause a range of physical and emotional symptoms, including hot flushes, mood swings and vaginal dryness.

The aim of HRT is to restore the level of these hormones, allowing the body to function normally again.

THE ROLE OF OESTROGEN

Oestrogen is known as the female hormone because it controls much of what makes women different from men – such as releasing eggs from ovaries.

Apart from regulating menstruation and playing a part in conception, it also plays a part in other functions such as healthy bones, skin temperature and moisture (particularly the vagina) and sex drive.

When that hormone reduces, the symptoms of a lack of oestrogen include hot flushes, night sweats, loss of libido, vaginal dryness and also bladder problems such as leaking urine when you cough or sneeze.

The oestrogen that is used in traditional HRT is taken from plants or the urine of pregnant horses.

THE ROLE OF PROGESTERONE

The main role of progesterone is to prepare the womb for pregnancy – while it also helps to protect the lining of the womb, or the endometrium.

Decreased levels don't have the same effect as a lack of oestrogen but it is recommended that progesterone is taken as well as oestrogen as part of hormone replacement therapy, as oestrogen on its own has been shown to increase the chances of womb, or endometrial cancer.

A synthetic form is usually added to the oestrogen supplements in HRT – although this is not needed in anyone who has had their womb removed.

THE TYPES OF HRT

Because women who have had a hysterectomy don't usually require progesterone – its main function being to protect the lining of the womb, they are generally prescribed oestrogen-only HRT

Those women suffering from menopausal symptoms but still have their periods are often prescribed cyclical HRT:

Monthly: This is where you would take oestrogen daily and progesterone for just the last two weeks of your cycle.

Three Monthly: There is also a three monthly version of cyclical HRT where you would take oestrogen daily but would take progesterone for two weeks at the end of a 13 week cycle, instead of each month. This is usually for women with irregular periods and is often encouraged so that regular bleeding is maintained, so the last period can be marked for the benefit of knowing when menopause can be diagnosed – i.e. one year from the date of the last period.

Continuous: For those women who are already at that stage – known as post-menopausal – then a continuous combined HRT is usually recommended.

This involves taking a combination of oestrogen and progestogen every day without any break.

TAKING HRT

Doctors tend to recommend a low dose of hormones at the start of treatment, to ensure that any side effects are minimal. If they don't have the desired effect then the dosage can be increased at a later date although the NHS Choices website suggests waiting a few months to see if the original prescription works. If not, they recommend talking to your GP who may consider changing the type of treatment you are on, or increasing the dose.

There are a great variety of ways to take HRT but generally they come in tablet form, taken by mouth, or as patches which can be stuck to your skin or an implant where small pellets of oestrogen are inserted under the skin – usually on the arm on tummy area. Some people also opt for gels which can be applied to the skin and absorbed.

Local oestrogen can also be used for vaginal dryness – a common problem in the menopause as the skin becomes thinner and the walls of the vagina become more sensitive. If this is the only symptom you have then the local treatment may be all that is required. This can be found in the form of pessaries, a vaginal ring or creams.

How long does the treatment last?

The guideline has been that two to five years – to see women through the symptoms of the menopause – is sufficient, although there are many incidents of people staying on HRT for much shorter, or longer, terms.

When coming off it, doctors recommend taking it slowly and decreasing doses gradually rather than just stopping overnight. This will help with a relapse into symptoms – which may still occur for a couple of months regardless.

Should you stop and the symptoms return for more than a few months then it is possible you can go back on HRT – or just look for other treatments for vaginal dryness and osteoporosis if they are the main concerns.

IS HRT FOR EVERYONE?

There has been much debate over recent years about the safety of HRT and after a few scares about increased cancer risk it became unpopular as a treatment of choice for the menopause.

This view is changing now and new research suggests that in many cases the benefits of HRT can outweigh the possible risks. This will depend on a number of factors; however, you may not be suitable to take it if you have:

- A history of breast cancer, ovarian cancer or womb cancer
- A history of blood clots
- A history of heart disease or stroke
- Untreated high blood pressure – your blood pressure will need to be controlled before you can start HRT
- Liver disease

SIDE EFFECTS OF HORMONE TREATMENT

For some people there are a few side effects of taking HRT and the severity can depend on dosage as well as sensitivity. If they persist for more than three months, take medical advice although initially you may experience:

BLEEDING

Often the progesterone element of the HRT can induce a monthly bleed in about 85% of women, particularly with the continuous combined versions. This is quite normal – certainly for the first six months - unless it becomes heavy or irregular in which case it should be reported to your GP.

FLUID RETENTION

Fluid retention and weight gain can go hand in hand, with increased incidence of bloating and swelling – particularly around the ankles, face and breasts, which can cause some tenderness. Many women fear putting on weight at this time but it can be other factors rather than the HRT – such as water retention but also decreased amounts of activity at this age.

It is thought that breast tenderness can be helped by Oil of Evening Primrose although if the problem persists for more than a few months it might be worth looking at changing the dose or type of HRT.

NAUSEA

Nausea associated with HRT can be reduced by taking tablets at night with food instead of morning or by changing from pill form to gels or patches.

BENEFITS AND RISKS

There have been many studies into HRT, with differing results. Some have warned of increased risks, particularly regarding breast cancer, while others have identified some very positive protection offered by the treatment.

Dr John C Stevenson is a specialist in heart disease as well as an expert in the impact the menopause has on women. In a recent report on Women's Health, written with Kate Maclaran, he said it has long been recognised that oestrogen protects against certain type of heart disease.

He added that the theory HRT offers protection against cardiovascular disease is well supported – despite the controversy that arose following publication of the Women's Health Initiative data which claimed the replacement therapy increased the risk of breast cancer – and even heart issues.

'Despite initial reports of excess cardiovascular harm with HRT subsequent analyses have shown that any increased risk is confined to older women or those further from menopause.'

The report states that the menopause is a pivotal time for reducing future cardiovascular risk and many women will seek medical help at this stage.

'It should be seen as an important opportunity to implement disease prevention strategies through dietary and lifestyle changes along with pharmacological measures if necessary.'

The report also states that in the future we should be seeing development of new treatments that have cardiovascular benefit but avoid any adverse effects on breast tissue or the womb lining.

Whatever the future holds, the main benefit for anyone suffering from menopausal symptoms is that HRT is a very effective solution, offering control over the worst symptoms and making a significant difference to a woman's quality of life and wellbeing.

HRT can also reduce a woman's risk of developing osteoporosis and cancer of the colon and rectum. However, long-term use is rarely recommended, and the NHS does warn that bone density will decrease rapidly after HRT is stopped.

As John Stevenson's report suggests, there is a slightly increased risk of developing breast cancer when taking the combined version – as well as similarly raised incidents – albeit marginal - of womb and ovarian cancers and strokes.

Studies into systemic HRT shows there is also an increase in the risk of deep vein thrombosis (DVT) and pulmonary embolism – a blockage in the pulmonary artery.

Another risk, often overlooked, is that of unwanted pregnancy. Although oestrogen is used in HRT it isn't as powerful as that used in the contraceptive pill and so it is possible to become pregnant while taking it. Some women can still be fertile for up to two years after her last period, particularly if she is under 50.

Many menopausal women on HRT opt for an intrauterine device – an IUS – which can act as the progesterone part of HRT while taking an oestrogen only supplement.

According to the NHS Choices website, most experts agree that if HRT is used on a short-term basis (no more than five years), the benefits outweigh the risks.

This is certainly the opinion of John Stevenson who said in a report into osteoporosis, written with T E J Stevenson: 'It has become quite clear that the initial safety concerns raised over ten years ago about HRT having major adverse effects have not been substantiated, and the risks of HRT are actually extremely small. It has also emerged that the alternative remedies all carry their own risks which are significant, if not more so, than those of HRT.'

He went on to say that for the prevention of post-menopausal osteoporosis, 'it is obvious that HRT should again become the first-line therapy, and the regulatory authorities must act to correct their advice.'

What The GP Can Offer

One of the possible ports of call for those women who have struggled with the menopause is often to see their GP. This may be the first port, or may be a last resort having exhausted all the alternative and lifestyle options available.

There is no harm in voicing your concerns. Often women present to their doctor with symptoms they don't relate to the menopause. This can often be digestive disorders, heart problems (palpitations) or general issues with sleeping, tiredness and so on.

It is always worth getting these kinds of symptoms checked out regardless because sometimes they can relate to other issues such as IBS, stress or a low functioning thyroid. It is likely that a GP would want to rule out all other issues with a blood test before categorically diagnosing the menopause.

On the basis that the symptoms are due to the change of life, what options can the GP offer to help alleviate symptoms?

One option could be HRT and it is important to look at the facts and risks. It is a useful method of reducing symptoms and many women have been amazed by its efficacy.

John C. Stevenson, the specialist previously mentioned. studies the effects of the menopause on women's health, Based at the Royal Brompton Hospital in London, he has a large number of patients who've been on HRT for many years with no adverse side effects – and who are determined to stay on it as long as possible.

All medical practitioners would advise looking into individual health factors before making any decisions and they are usually very willing to discuss the issues, and latest research, with their patients.

The GP might offer HRT or ERT – the oestrogen only version – because it is often seen as the first line of treatment for reducing menopausal symptoms.

The most popular treatment is tablet form because of the ease of changing prescription if necessary, and usually starts with a low does. If higher doses are required, these are usually achieved with an implant. For short term use of three to six months, it may be that a vaginal cream or pessary treatment will be sufficient.

Patches are also convenient to use and are popular – particularly since the material used now is kinder to the skin and causes less skin irritation than previous versions, which had higher alcohol content.

Implants tend to only be prescribed at the time of hysterectomy and ovarian removal and provide gradually decreasing levels of oestrogen over a few months. They need replacing on a regular basis but can help those who might forget to take pills.

Treatment is now also available through a nasal spray – said to give relief for up to 24 hours although some women don't like the effect the spray has on their throat and nose. Gels and creams are also a possibility although doctors can be wary of prescribing them because of the difficulty in prescribing the exact dose.

Often HRT treatments can take 3-6 months to become fully effective but don't be worried about returning to your doctor to get further advice if you feel there is something wrong, particularly unusual bleeding or extensive side effects. There are many types of HRT and it may just be a case of trying more than one to get the right type to suit you.

For some women, HRT is unsuitable – whether because of a hormone related illness or because it causes too many side effects. Those likely to be considered unsuitable would be those who have:

- Unexplained vaginal bleeding.
- Active breast cancer.
- Liver disease.

- Endometriosis – this condition may be reactivated by HRT
- Fibroids – the hormones can cause bleeding
- Women prone to forming blood clots.

In these cases there are other medicines that the doctor might consider prescribing. There are a number of new drugs that target hormonal problems and give significant relief, but without the risks or problems that can be associated with traditional hormone therapy.

TIBOLONE

Tibolone is a synthetic steroid used to treat many menopausal symptoms, with the added benefit of helping to prevent bone loss. Tibolone is also reported as being able to improve mood without affecting the breast or uterine tissues. Tibolone is not suitable if you are experiencing symptoms of the menopause before it actually starts (known as the peri-menopause) or within a year of your last period.

RALOXIFENE

Raloxifene is what is known as a SERM - Selective Estrogen Receptor Modulator – which copies the action of oestrogen in some tissues while blocking it in others. It also helps improve mood and is licensed for the treatment of osteoporosis.

ANTIDEPRESSANTS

There are a host of different drugs that come under the headings of SSRIs (Selective serotonin reuptake inhibitors) and SNRI (serotonin and noradrenaline reuptake inhibitors) which not only helps mood but also the incidents of hot flushes. They aren't designed for the menopause but are often prescribed because of their ability to control flushing.

SSRIs include paroxetine, fluoxetine, escitalopram and citalopram while venlafaxine is an SNRI and has also been shown to reduce hot flushes almost immediately.

They can have side-effects such as nausea and reduced libido but are deemed to be safer for women than HRT in some cases.

GABAPENTIN

Gabapentin is a drug that is usually used to control epileptic seizures and pain. However, research has shown that it eases menopausal flushing symptoms in some women.

CLONIDINE

Clonidine is a medicine originally designed to treat high blood pressure, but research shows it may reduce hot flushes and night sweats in some menopausal women.

Clonidine can cause unpleasant side effects, including dry mouth, drowsiness, depression, constipation and fluid retention.

You will need to take it for a trial period of two to four weeks, to test its effectiveness. If your symptoms don't improve during this time, or if you experience any side effects, the treatment should be stopped and you should go back to your GP.

A list of drugs you might come across to treat menopausal symptoms include:

- **Venlafaxine: (Effexor®)**
  There can be temporary side effects such as nausea and also high blood pressure if on a high dose. This is one of the drugs offered for women taking tamoxifen and therefore not suited to HRT.
- **Desvenlafaxine: (Pristiq®)**
  The side effects can be similar to venlafaxine and fluoxetine. Thought to be useful in terms of controlling hot flushes.
- **Fluoxetine: (Prozac®)**
  Side effects similar to those above, plus lower libido and insomnia. Improvement in hot flushes has been shown in well-designed studies. Not suitable for women taking tamoxifen.

- **Paroxetine: (Paxil®)**
  Side effects as above. Rated to be best for dealing with hot flushes and sleep issues.
- **Escitalopram: (Lexapro®)**
  As above but can also induce an abnormal EKG. Thought to be good for dealing with hot flushes.
- **Gabapentin: (Neurontin®)**
  Side effects can be tiredness and lethargy, dizziness, weight gain, nausea and swelling. Mainly a treatment for insomnia.
- **Clonidine: (Catapres®)**
  Can cause a dry mouth, drowsiness, fatigue, constipation. It can lower blood pressure. Mainly used for hot flushes.

Over The Counter

GELS AND HYDRATION

Carrie Osman and her partners couldn't believe how limited the options were when it came to intimate care – which is why they set up SASS, a brand that deals specifically with vaginal dryness.

'Whilst digging into data we found that although some 3 million women going through the menopause were suffering with symptoms such as vaginal dryness, a huge 75% of women in the UK were suffering in silence.'

She added that vaginal dryness can have such a major impact on women's lives, preventing them from enjoying their life as they want to, leaving them feeling out of control and sometimes anxious.

'Many women express this as feeling 'hindered'. The reality was that a high proportion of women didn't feel there was any answer to this 'unspoken' issue. At SASS we didn't believe that anyone should feel held back by intimate issues. We wanted to create a product that women could use with ease and feel comfortable buying.'

They started off by producing their Intimate Dryness Gel - created so it can be applied manually to provide immediate, long lasting intimate hydration and relief.

Whilst developing their first product, they began to understand more about the needs of 'the intimate area' and the SASS pH Balanced Serum came to life.

'There are lots of everyday things that can cause microbial imbalances – tight jeans, exercise, sexual activity etc. This serum soothes, calms and rebalances irritated skin. One woman who got in touch told us that the pH Balanced Serum is life changing and that she had given up hope, while another going through early menopause had thought her sex life was over for good before she discovered SASS.'

Social worker Melanie Parkinson is one person who calls the SASS serum 'a miracle cure'. She claimed there were times she thought her sex life was over for good.

'It was frightening. I'd always had a very healthy sex drive and then overnight down below became a no-go area. It was awful. 'I had literally tried everything and felt like giving up but this serum has given me my old life back. 'I never thought the answer would be in a little £12 tube on sale in Boots.

She had tried HRT but she kept suffering repeated bouts of severe thrush, which left her uncomfortable down below – adding to problems with her sex life.

'This miracle serum has given me my sex life back and I feel like the old me again,' said Melanie.

The team at SASS have since developed a full range of intimate skin care that is pH balanced and tested and approved by gynaecologists.

There are a number of other lubricants and moisturisers on the market – KY Jelly and Vagisil both being available over the counter.

SLEEPWEAR

There are a variety of different types of sleepwear to help women deal with night sweats which end up soaking clothes and sheets while in bed – which can then lead to cold, shivering and being unable to sleep. Fabric brands include Coolmax ® and also Intera ®

BEDDING

As well as moisture wicking clothing, many women also opt for specific bedding products to help with night sweats.

The aim is to treat the sleeping surface rather than the body – so that as moisture evaporates, the subsequent wetness and hot flushing are reduced.

Again the technology relies on structured fibres that create thin channels to wick moisture away and dry skin more quickly, preventing friction with the skin.

GEL PADS

Similarly to the aim of specific bedding, gel pads to place under sheets contain a substance that transfers heat away from the body.

When held against pulse points, such as the wrists, the pad will gently cool your blood as it passes through your body and lower your temperature. A cool surface can help relieve aching, tired muscles; it can soothe a throbbing headache and help to reduce inflammation. These pads can be used to sleep or rest on when feeling symptoms, and are particularly noted for helping with the immediate relief of hot flushes.

A variety of sizes are usually available so that they can be used on beds but also sofas or chairs, or even inside pillows.

SUPPLEMENTS

There are many supplements devised specifically for the menopause that include some or all of the herbs, vitamins and natural remedies mentioned throughout this book.

Research carried out by the The Good Housekeeping Institute showed that two supplements can lessen the side effects of menopause: black cohosh and soy isoflavones (from soybean or red clover sources). It also warned that women should look out for excessive doses as they can be counter-productive and possibly even dangerous.

It is also worth remembering that some herbal supplements, such as St John's Wort, can interact with other drugs so care needs to be taken when considering taking anything that isn't approved by a doctor if you are taking any other kind of medication.

Complementary and Alternative Therapies

The combination of concerns about HRT and increased awareness of alternative medicine means that more and more women are looking to methods other than prescription solutions to their menopause symptoms.

Whether used alone or in conjunction with more traditional remedies, all seem to have their place in terms of helping to alleviate symptoms.

Research is always recommended – as is seeking treatment from practitioners who are registered with their own governing bodies, or who have been recommended by a registered health expert.

Although there are some warnings, as with any therapies, most are considered to be unlikely to cause any harm – and many are reporting excellent results with the physical and emotional issues of the change of life.

ACUPUNCTURE

Tamzin Freeman is a London-based therapist with a particular interest in menopause, using a range of treatments including acupuncture, which she explains is part of Traditional Chinese Medicine.

'It works on the basis that energy, or qi (pronounced "chee"), runs through the body along channels called meridians - illness occurs when that flow is disrupted. Acupuncture stimulates precise points on the meridians to restore balance and a healthy flow of energy.'

She added that scientists are starting to identify some of the physiological mechanisms at work, and there's evidence that the insertion of needles into designated acupuncture points speeds the conduction of electromagnetic signals within the body. These signals may increase the flow of endorphins and other pain-relieving chemicals, as well as immune system cells, which aid healing.

It is Tamzin's main treatment for menopausal symptoms because she finds it effective although she believes it needs regular treatment.

'It helps with the hot flushes (caused by Yin deficiency), mood swings, insomnia, headaches and tiredness', she said – citing one of her patients who came to see her with really poor energy levels.

'Melissa was suffering from really low energy, bad sweats, insomnia, aches on waking on rising, and a very strong appetite.'

Her periods had been erratic and she felt really teary. Her skin was "like sand paper" with little bumps.

Following her first treatment Melissa told Tamzin she'd got "the most awful headache" which lasted about 24 hours. Following the headache, her energy levels improved to 7/10, and the stiffness in the morning was much better. Appetite was less strong, but the sweats hadn't really changed.

After five weekly treatments her energy had improved greatly and the sweats, aches, skin, appetite and mood were all improved to some level.

ALEXANDER TECHNIQUE

The aim of this therapy is to allow good breathing to help energy flow, creating 'postural harmony' which gives freedom to the mind and spirit. Although there is no evidence that the technique specifically helps menopausal symptoms, the breathing technique has been shown to reduce hot flushes by 39%.

AROMATHERAPY

When people think of aromatherapy, often they think of massage treatments.

It is true that the addition of essential oils to massage blends and other treatments can really help you through this difficult milestone of your life – but sometimes just smelling the oils can be enough to help take the edge of difficult symptoms.

Aromatherapy oils are used for their ability to help the body balance and regulate various systems and emotions and the ones most used for the menopause include:

- **Basil (Ocimumbasilicum)**
  For lack of concentration, poor energy, lethargy.
- **Chamomile Roman (Anthemisnobilis)**
  Used for sleep issues, aches and pains, headaches and skin problems.
- **Clary sage (Salvia sclarea)**
  Helps to regulate sweat glands and so is good for dealing with hot flushes, sweating, insomnia, disturbed sleep patterns.
- **Cypress (Cupressussempervirens)**
  This is most known for its ability to relieve fluid retention, hot flushes, and mood swings.
- **Geranium (Pelargonium graveolens)**
  Good for irritability and depression and for alleviating the problem of dry skin.
- **Peppermint (Menthapiperita)**
  For digestion, hot flushes, sweating, headaches, fatigue.

You don't have to book a massage session to get the benefit of aromatherapy (although this is a great thing to do as massage, alone, is great for easing tension.)

One of the most common ways of getting essential oils into the body is by having a warm bath – with 6-8 drops of your chosen oil added to the water. The oils can be mixed up to deal with a range of symptoms and it is recommended to stay in the bath for at least thirty minutes to get the true benefits.

You can also use diluted oils – at a ratio of around two per cent in almond oil – for massage, (about 5 drops to 10ml of almond oil) – or you can add a similar amount to a body lotion applying it after a shower.

To help relieve symptoms while on the go, essential oils can be inhaled directly from a tissue or you can put them in a diffuser or burner around the house or office.

One recommendation for hot flushes or a headache is to inhale peppermint essential oil – soaked into a tissue – at the first sign of either.

For stress and depression try these techniques with geranium, lavender, grapefruit, camomile, bergamot and/or neroli essential oils.

AYERVEDA

Ayerveda is an Indian form of treatment which brings together all aspects a person in terms of their health. Known as the 'Science of Life', wellness is determined from an examination of the pulse and nails.

Treatments can include massage as well as cleansing treatments such as enemas, coupled with herb treatment and dietary advice.

HOMEOPATHY

Homeopathy aims to promote wellbeing by encouraging the body's own natural healing capacity.

With the menopause, homeopathy doesn't treat different symptoms but treats everything within the body, believing them all to be interconnected. So if going for a consultation expect to be treated as a 'whole' person and not just as a list of symptoms.

Homeopathic practitioners claim their remedies for menopause are safe – mainly because very small amounts of the active ingredients are used in their preparation.

Unlike herbal medicine, homeopathic remedies come from a variety of sources including plants but also minerals, metals and even some poisons – most of which have been routinely used for hundreds of years.

The following are most likely to be used for women suffering with the menopause:

- **Lachesis**
  Prepared from the venom of a South American snake, this remedy is used for a general feeling of malaise as well as any bleeding, fainting, weakness, sadness, irregular periods, hormonal fluctuations, hot flushes, palpitations, headaches, nausea.

- **Sepia**
  Sepia – also known as the 'washer-woman's remedy', because people who need this remedy tend to be tired and emotional and with a sharp tongue, particularly towards loved ones. Prepared from cuttlefish ink the remedy is often used with sulphuric acid.

- **Sulphuric Acid**
  This remedy is just what it says it is and is used to deal with digestive weakness, flushing, irritability and a general feeling of impatience and anxiety that can accompany the menopause.

- **Folliculinum**
  This treatment is thought to be good for many symptoms of the menopause including restlessness, dizziness, weight problems, food cravings, flooding, hot flushes, vaginal dryness and fibroids. It is also thought to help restore clarity.

- **Calcium Carbonicum**
  Made from oyster shells, this is the traditional treatment for anxiety and worry although it is also useful for dealing with hot flushes and perspiration.

- **Pulsatilla**
  This remedy, made from the windflower, helps to deal with irregular and/or painful periods as well as difficult sleeping, hot flushes and restless legs.

EFT

EFT is described by its founder, Gary Craig, as a "psychological form of acupuncture" - mentally focusing on a physical or emotional issue whilst tapping on various acupuncture points - so, it can work on both physical and emotional issues.

With regard to the menopause it can be used to address emotional issues, either of the change of life itself, or other issues which feel much worse because of the emotional instability of the menopause.

HYPNOSIS

Scientists in the US have undertaken studies showing that hot flushes can be reduced by as much as 75 per cent using hypnosis. According to the research at the University of Texas and Baylor University, women reporting this significant improvement had five hypnosis sessions per week.

The study, published in the journal Menopause, was the first of its kind and reported that the women were given suggestions for mental images of coolness, a safe place or relaxation, depending on their preference. They also received an audio recording of a hypnotic induction and were asked to listen to it each day. A second group of women met with a doctor five times a week to talk about their symptoms – and they also received an audio recording, but it contained information about hot flushes.

Twelve weeks later, the hypnosis group was found to have had 75 per cent fewer hot flushes, compared with 13 per cent who saw a doctor. The hypnosis group also reported an 80 per cent decrease in frequency and severity of the hot flushes; this was only 15 per cent for other women.

Also, the hypnosis group reported being able to sleep better and have less disruption in their lives compared with the control group.

Researchers suggested the results were such because of the fact hypnosis can boost the function of the parasympathetic nerve system, which plays a part in how the body heats up during flushing.

REFLEXOLOGY

Dating back to Ancient Egypt, reflexology is the practice of treating reflex points and areas in the feet and hands that relate to corresponding parts of the body.

Each organ and structure within the body is linked to the feet by energy channels or meridians. When ill or stressed, our physical or emotional health is weakened and these channels can become blocked. Reflexology can be used very effectively to restore the free flow of energy and therefore bring the body back to a state of health.

Research carried out at the UK School of Complementary Health in Exeter produced some very positive results in terms of the efficacy of this treatment – indicating a noticeable decrease in anxiety, depression, insomnia, hot flushes and night sweats among menopausal women who received regular reflexology over a 4 month period.

Reflexologist, Sarah Finley, MIRI, says on her website that during menopause, reflexology works by regulating the hormones and glandular functions of the body.

'It can help to alleviate and balance both the physical and emotional systems. By working with the hypothalamus and pituitary, reflexology can help to restore balance to the endocrine system. This in turn can alleviate menopausal symptoms such as hot flushes as well as mood swings and anxiety,'

She adds that by calming the central nervous system, sleep disturbances can also be alleviated and anxiety and stress levels reduced. By regulating calcium and phosphorous levels in the thyroid gland, bone loss can prevented. Reflexology also helps the ovaries to regulate their oestrogen secretions and the uterus to maintain its natural health and flexibility.

The effects of reflexology are cumulative and, depending on specific needs and symptoms, a course of treatments is usually recommended.

REIKI

Reiki healing originated in Japan and is a non-invasive healing treatment. Meaning 'universal life energy' it works by helping the body to repair itself by balancing the energy system of the body.

During a reiki session, the practitioner can either work 'hands off' so you don't feel them at all, or they will place their hands in various patterns on the body using very light touches.

The aim is to channel positive energy into the body, to encourage health and healing. It is thought to be beneficial to menopausal women because it is known to help balance the different systems in the body, including the hormonal system, therefore helping with menstrual cycles, migraines and hot flushes.

TAI CHI

Tai chi is an ancient Chinese marital art that combines mind and body therapy into one healing practice.

It involves an awareness of breathing coupled with a series of low-impact, slow motion movements – often named after animal movements such as 'snake creeps down'.

There have been a number of studies that show tai chi's ability to alleviate the many symptoms of menopause, particularly problems associated with bone loss, anxiety and depression. The gentle movements help to develop relaxed muscles without putting any strain on joints or connective tissues – making it ideal for anyone with limiting health conditions.

Tai chi is thought to help with osteoporosis – and the problems associated with it – by giving a better sense of our body within space while also developing muscle strength and flexibility. Recent studies show that people who regularly practice the art – five times a week for 45 minutes or more – slowed the rate of bone loss by around three times, against a control group of postmenopausal women who did not partake in tai chi.

YOGA

The discipline of yoga promotes stretching, deep breathing and relaxation which can have an effect on how well a woman will cope with menopausal changes. It focuses on improving well-being rather than specifically controlling symptoms but is reported to be useful for dealing with stress and anxiety.

Herbal Medicines

Many people who are concerned about taking prescription medication for the menopause often turn to alternative methods of controlling the symptoms of the menopause.

One popular source of help comes from the wide variety of herbal medicines available.

These are derived from natural sources – although it should be noted that the vast majority of prescription and over-the-counter medications are also from such sources and therefore all need to be treated with respect. Natural doesn't always mean safe. This is particularly the case for women being treated for certain cancers, as phytoestrogens can have the effect of blocking certain drugs such as Tamoxifen – used to treat those who have had breast cancer.

If you do use herbal supplements it is advised to keep your doctor informed, should they interact with any other treatments – whether for the menopause or not.

Some women claim that GPs can be cautious about endorsing or embracing most herbal supplements – and this tends to be because there have been few controlled studies in this area. However, more and more medical practitioners are working to better understand herbal therapies so they are sufficiently informed to offer advice.

Warnings aside, many herbal remedies go back centuries and have time-honoured favour among herbal medicine practitioners.

For example, black cohosh has a long history of use at the time of the menopause. The herb is native to North America and is thought to be useful in combatting hot flushes and night sweats, although HRT supporters will say it doesn't help with cardiac or bone health.

It is part of the buttercup family and it is the root of the plant that is used – not least because it contains a complex mix of natural chemicals which some claim are as potent as many modern drugs.

Sage is another herb that has gained great popularity for its ability to calm hot flushes and night sweats – possibly because it directly decreases the production of sweat.

Sage is rich in essential oils and this is the reason it gives off a strong scent. These oils also form an important part in the plant's medicinal function. Today, sage extracts are well known and widely used for their ability to help relieve the symptoms of menopausal sweats and hot flushes.

TV news reader, Carol Barnes, said that it was sage that sorted out her menopausal issues. In an interview with the Daily Mail online she said she had been to see her doctor, who'd put her on HRT.

She said it was before all the cancer scares and she said her symptoms did get better – her hot flushes and sweating had gone and her libido came back.

However HRT caused her to get very heavy periods and although she stayed on HRT for six years, once the negative reports came in she decided to come off it.

'Sure enough, as I came off the HRT the symptoms returned, but now I was also getting night sweats, which would leave me drenched in perspiration,' she said.

So, she did some research and decided to try out some natural remedies to help alleviate the flushes.

She took sage which she claims was 'incredible' and that after just a week her hot flushes and sweating went. 'It also seemed to help with all the other symptoms. I slept better, probably because I no longer had the night sweats, and it seemed to put me on an even keel mood-wise. '

Despite being well past the menopause now, she keeps taking Sage as she believes it is now good for other things, such as keeping her memory healthy.

Agnus Castus is also known as Vitex Agnus castus or Chaste berry. Extracts obtained from the berries of the plant have a long history of use for treating menstrual symptoms in women still having their monthly cycle.

More recent research suggests its popularity in past centuries is well placed, not least because the berries of this plant modify the hormonal balance between oestrogen and progesterone – to the point it can bring back periods once they start faltering, regulate heavy periods and also restoring fertility when caused by hormonal imbalance. Strangely enough, though, taken in excess it can mimic one of the lesser known menopausal symptoms of 'crawling skin' and so care is advised in terms of dosage. The herb should not be used at the same time as other prescribed hormonal medicines such as HRT or the oral contraceptive pill.

St. John's Wort has been shown, in some cases, to be more effective than prescription drugs for treating depression – one of the symptoms regularly reported during menopause. Recent trials revealed that the herb, when taken in doses less than 1.2mg per day, produced a 61% improvement in mild to moderate depression – while higher doses generated even better responses.

The name of St John's Wort (Hypericumperforatum) is said to have arisen from the fact that it is in full bloom and traditionally harvested on St John's day – the 24th of June.

One of the side effects which needs to be considered – particularly for those working outside or living in sunny environments – is that the herb can cause light sensitivity so exposure to sun should be avoided.

It is also not recommended for those on the contraceptive pill, taking anti-epilepsy treatments and a number of other drugs - including anti-depressants.

Dong Quai is a traditional Chinese medicine and is sometimes called the female ginseng, often used to treat menopausal symptoms. Also known as Angelica sinensis it is known both in China and the

West for its ability to support and maintain the natural balance of female hormones. It does not have any oestrogen effect and it is one of the herbs for menopause that should not be taken if a woman is experiencing heavy bleeding.

Wild Yam is the base for pharmaceutical progesterone and although a great source for this hormone it can't be produced without a complicated conversion process, in a laboratory. Often this causes confusion and women cannot rely on supplements of this herb if they require progesterone.

Extracts of soy have been used for many years to support women through the menopause. They can be used at all stages of the menopause and is particularly useful when a woman experiences a broad range of symptoms such as tiredness, irritability, poor memory and a general feeling of not being oneself. Supplements made from fermented soya beans contain isoflavones which are absorbed better by the body and hence, work better.

Soy isoflavones can be used together with other herbs targeting specific symptoms – for instance, if hot flushes are particularly troublesome, use together with Sage. The isoflavones in soy foods help balance hormone levels and have some oestrogenic activity. There is on-going research about the safety and efficacy of isolated soy isoflavone supplements. Most practitioners recommend using natural soy foods rather than supplements. Choose from tofu, soy milk, roasted soy nuts or tempeh.

Valeriana has been used for many decades to treat stress and anxiety. The root is harvested as a drug that is used for settling the mind and relaxing the body, it is also used to help aid sleep – often disturbed during the menopause. In addition, valerian can be found in products designed for stress relief.

Devil's Claw grows in the Kalahari Desert, and pretty much nowhere else. It gets its name from the claw-like fruit produced by the plant. However, it is not the fruit, but the root of Devil's Claw

(Harpagophytumprocumbens) that is used by women suffering from menopausal pains in muscles and joints.

Often the menopause is diagnosed around the same time as women are likely to suffer from a low acting or underactive thyroid. This is where kelp, or sea kelp, is often recommended by herbal practitioners. The group of plants, also known as brown algae contain iodine and as such have specific properties. Iodine is a substance that is essential for normal thyroid function which in turn, helps the body maintain a healthy weight and vitality.

Sea kelp is also used in many cultures as a food not only for its benefits to the activity of the thyroid but also as a well-known treatment for thinning hair. Menopausal women often complain of hair loss, thinning hair and a general lack of lustre, which kelps claims to revive. Millet has similar properties, being a good source of silicon – an essential trace element for strength and structure of hair.

Ginkgo Biloba is one of the most researched herbs and as such we now know that it plays a strong part in maintaining normal blood circulation, particularly to the brain. This helps concentration and memory, both of which seem to fail to some degree during the menopause.

A Ginkgo biloba tree is said to have survived the bombing of Hiroshima at the end of World War 2. This resilience has not gone unnoticed by those who believe that ginkgo is amongst our most valuable herbs for people in mid to old age.

Other recommended supplements include flaxseed, which contain substances called lignins -important modulators of hormone metabolism. Some people grind it up and use one or two tablespoons a day in their food – such as on top of cereals or in soups.

Vitamin E is said to help with hot flushes if taken at a daily dose of around 400 IUs while B vitamins may help women deal with the stress brought about by many symptoms of the menopause.

Evening primrose oil or black currant oil are both sources of gamma-linolenic acid (GLA), an essential fatty acid that can help influence prostaglandin synthesis and help moderate menopausal symptoms.

While many women, concerned about differing reports regarding HRT, have turned to herbal medicines, there are still some worries being stated by the medical profession.

They say that just because a product is labelled 'natural' does not mean that it is automatically safe and free from potentially damaging chemicals.

A recent guideline from the National Institute for Health and Care Excellence (NICE) Clinical Knowledge Summaries states that "CKS does not recommend the use of complementary therapies". The reasons include:

- They have not been shown convincingly to work very well.
- There is very little control over the quality of the products available, which may vary.
- Some of these treatments have properties similar to oestrogen and should not be used in women who should not take oestrogen (for example, women with breast cancer).
- Long-term safety (for example, effects on the breast and lining of the womb (uterus)) have not been assessed.
- Some may have serious side-effects. For example, severe liver damage has been reported – albeit rarely - with black cohosh.
- Some herbs contain chemicals called coumarins, which make them unsuitable if you take anticoagulants (such as warfarin).

The Last Word

OK, so hopefully I've covered a range of options for ways of dealing with the menopause.

But I can't get away from the fact I was inspired to write this book because of my passion for magnetic therapy and how it has worked not only for me, but for many hundreds of my clients who ring regularly to tell me how their life has changed.

Magnetic therapy has been used for many years and is thought to enhance the natural process of healing, perhaps by improvement in circulation, an effect on nerve signals or a change in cells involved in healing – but it still isn't recognised in medical fields.

A national survey of 508 women in 2006, showed a significant reduction in symptoms when using a magnet designed to help with the menopause. No side effects were reported.

There are a number of scientific facts available to support why this is the case.

For example, it is thought that magnets help ease symptoms during the menopause – by helping rebalance the Autonomic Nervous System (ANS).

The natural reduction in hormones through menopause cause an imbalance to the ANS, which is responsible for controlling bodily functions, including stress reactions such as sweating, body temperature, circulation, heart rate, bowel and bladder function, and more.

There are two divisions of the ANS, the Sympathetic Nervous system (SNS) and the Parasympathetic Nervous System (PNS). The SNS controls symptoms such as sweating and anxiety while the PNS is responsible for repair and digestion – the opposite.

The current thinking is that the power of the magnets brings the two divisions into unison and helps the body balance itself to reduce symptoms – by reducing excessive sympathetic nervous system (SNS) activity and increasing parasympathetic activity.

That's the science bit, but what is clear is the number of people who claim they work. They don't need to know why – they are just pleased to have their life back.

No, you're not going Bonkers.

You're just going through puberty, backwards.

Enjoy the ride!

Please visit my website for further details about me & Aura^3

www.aura3.co.uk

The Aura^3 website provides detailed information on Magnetic Therapy and also offers the opportunity to browse and shop the extensive range of Energetix Jewellery and well-being products for Women, Men, Children and pets.

You can also find my full range of cosmetic products 'Sheila's Natural Creams & Balms' through the Aura^3 website.

Sheila's Natural Creams & Balms have been developed to complement Aura^3's magnetic well-being products. Handmade from the finest ingredients nature has to offer, Sheila's Natural Products are paraben free, contain no petrochemical related ingredients, no SLS, no GM ingredients, are not tested on animals and wherever possible are completely organic. Plus they are lovingly made in the UK.

My mission is to constantly strive to expand the Aura^3 range and provide Natural and alternative products suitable for women of all ages so please do keep in touch.

You can follow Aura^3 on Facebook and Twitter

Facebook: Aura3uk

Twitter: @aura3uk

Or you can follow me personally via
Facebook: SheilaWenborne
Twitter: @sheilawenborne

Or keep up to date with my new ventures, news and appearances via
the website
www.sheilawenborne.com

Acknowledgements

I would like to say a huge thank you to all of the following people, as without their help and support this book could never have been written.

JOE WENBORNE
My Tin Hat wearing husband, for his constant love, support and encouragement.

PAT SMITH
My darling, long suffering mother. Thank you for giving birth to me, let's face it, without you I wouldn't be here…Thanks mum.

JANET KELLY
Without her hard work, incredible research and wealth of knowledge, this would have been little more than a colouring book.

EMMA DYOS
Who's been there from the start and worked tirelessly to make this happen.   Thanks for sticking with me and never giving up.

MURRAY HARKIN
My darling friend who started this journey with me back in April 2015 and has introduced me to a whole new world.

CLARE NORDBRUCH

My technical and creative wizard. Thanks Clare for dragging me kicking and screaming into the 21st Century. #YouareAmazing.

ANNIE POWELL

For your expertise and knowledge of natural products that has put Sheila's Natural Creams & Balms Range firmly on the map.

ROBERT DUNCAN

For bringing the words of this book to life with his amazing illustrations. Thank you Rob.

FINALLY

And last but not least, to 'Fearless Bob' my Border Collie who took me down the magnet therapy route along with the rest of my Collie family, Chip, Briney and our newest addition Mr. Wiggins. x

So... That's why I'm Bonkers! A Girl's guide to surviving the Menopause.
Sheila Wenborne

Printed in Great Britain
by Amazon